Fast Facts:
Contraception

Third edition

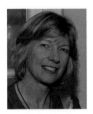

Ailsa E Gebbie MB ChB FRCOG FFSRH
Consultant Gynecologist
NHS Lothian Family Planning Services
Edinburgh
Scotland, UK

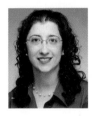

Katharine O'Connell White MD MPH FACOG
Assistant Clinical Professor
Department of Obstetrics and Gynecology
Columbia University
New York
NY, USA

Declaration of Independence
This book is as balanced and as practical as we can make it.
Ideas for improvement are always welcome: feedback@fastfacts.com

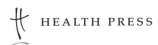

HEALTH PRESS

Fast Facts: Contraception
First published 2000; second edition 2005
Third edition February 2009

Text © 2009 Ailsa E Gebbie, Katharine O'Connell White
© 2009 in this edition Health Press Limited
Health Press Limited, Elizabeth House, Queen Street, Abingdon,
Oxford OX14 3LN, UK
Tel: +44 (0)1235 523233
Fax: +44 (0)1235 523238

Book orders can be placed by telephone or via the website.
For regional distributors or to order via the website, please go to:
www.fastfacts.com
For telephone orders, please call +44 (0)1752 202301 (UK and Europe),
1 800 247 6553 (USA, toll free), +1 419 281 1802 (Americas) or
+61 (0)2 9351 6173 (Asia–Pacific).

Fast Facts is a trademark of Health Press Limited.

A CIP record for this title is available from the British Library.

ISBN 978-1-905832-50-7

Gebbie, Ailsa E
Fast Facts: Contraception/
Ailsa E Gebbie and Katharine O'Connell White

Medical illustrations by Dee McLean, London, UK.
Typesetting and page layout by Zed, Oxford, UK.
Printed by Latimer Trend & Company Limited, Plymouth, UK.

Text printed with vegetable inks on biodegradable and
recyclable paper manufactured from sustainable forests.

Low
chlorine

Sustainable
forests

Glossary of abbreviations

BBT: basal body temperature

BMD: bone mineral density

COC: combined oral contraceptive

DMPA: depot medroxyprogesterone acetate

ED: every-day [preparation]

FAB: fertility-awareness-based [biological method]

FSH: follicle-stimulating hormone

HFI: hormone-free interval

HIV: human immunodeficiency virus

HPV: human papilloma virus

IUD: intrauterine device

LAM: lactational amenorrhea method

LARC: long-acting reversible contraceptive

LH: luteinizing hormone

LNG-IUS: levonorgestrel–intrauterine system

MI: myocardial infarction

PFI: pill-free interval

POP: progestogen-only pill

STI: sexually transmitted infection

VTE: venous thromboembolism

WHO: World Health Organization

Introduction

This is the third edition of *Fast Facts: Contraception*. On quick inspection, you would be forgiven for thinking that the past few years have seen relatively few new contraceptive methods emerge and little overall change in the areas of family planning and sexual health. This, however, masks the fact that huge initiatives have been taking place on both sides of the Atlantic to raise the profile of contraception, traditionally a rather Cinderella service, for it to become a thriving specialty encompassing all sexual and reproductive health issues.

Contraception and sexually transmitted infections (STIs) are now finally being managed in many fully integrated services. Common sense and logic has brought together the two specialties, which after all are both intimately concerned with sex!

Individuals who work in sexual health services are often passionate about their work and the issues that they deal with. They are often prepared to put their heads above the parapet and fight for the cause, particularly when health inequalities, women's rights and freedom of choice are at stake. Sexual health is a truly multidisciplinary specialty: the roles of nurses, pharmacists and other professionals have been extended and they are highly valued as hands-on providers.

Education means everything in life and poor educational attainment is an accurate predictor of reproductive health status. It determines your chance of teenage pregnancy, contracting an STI and having an abortion. One of the major roles of anyone working in sexual health is that of educator. Numerous guidelines now exist to lead evidence-based practice. However, for many professionals, time is very short and downloading weighty guidance documents is a step too far. We hope that this concise book will give practical and easy-to-read information to those working in primary care and as family physicians. If we have given you new information that can be directly translated into offering individuals a broader range of contraceptive options then we will feel writing this book has been a task well done.

1 Choosing a contraceptive method

Men and women will use contraception for many years, often over decades. Their needs will change over time; for example, what worked for a young woman during her years of education may be less appropriate once she is a busy working mother. Some individuals know exactly what method of contraception they want to use and require no medical assistance or only a brief appointment to obtain a prescription. However, many men and women are unaware of the full range of contraceptive options.

Decision-making may be daunting, so individuals will often look to healthcare professionals to help make sense of all the options. Whilst it is true that women take most of the responsibility for contraception, the needs and wishes of both partners must always be considered if contraception is to be used effectively.

Unintended pregnancy is common in both the UK and USA. Almost 50% of women who have an unintended pregnancy conceive while using no method of contraception; the other 50% report use of contraception in the month of conception but many have not used the method consistently or correctly.

It is important to remember that most contraceptive methods are possible options for most healthy women and, in general, the best method for a given woman is the method she chooses for herself. It is easy to over-medicalize contraception, particularly when the consultation is used as an opportunity for health screening, such as performing cervical (Pap) cytology. The prevalence of use of the common methods of contraception in the UK and USA is shown in Figure 1.1.

The consultation

When discussing contraception, there is much information to convey – and often not much time. The discussion about each method should cover mechanism of action, efficacy/effectiveness, benefits, risks, side effects and use of the method.

Ultimately, the aim is to allow the contraceptive user to make an informed choice of a method with which she feels confident and safe, and that she knows how to use correctly.

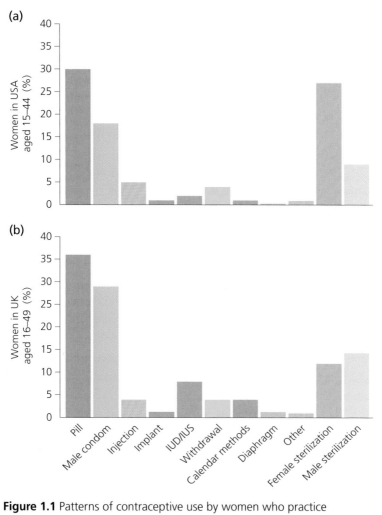

Figure 1.1 Patterns of contraceptive use by women who practice contraception: (a) aged 15–44 in the USA (2004); (b) aged 16–49 in the UK (2008). US data adapted from Vital and Health Statistics, Mosher et al. 2004; UK data adapted from the Office for National Statistics Omnibus Survey, Lader and Hopkins 2008. 'Other' includes female condom and spermicides. IUD/IUS, intrauterine device/system.

Mechanism of action. Women usually do not need to hear how oral contraceptives cause negative feedback in the hypothalamic–pituitary–ovarian axis, but they should have a basic understanding of how their contraceptive method works. Common misconceptions include thinking that oral contraceptive pills need only be taken at the time of intercourse, not realizing that the pill provides protection during the pill-free/placebo-pill time, and thinking the pill can be stopped when bleeding starts. A simple explanation of how a method of contraception works is always helpful and often helps dispel some of the misunderstandings surrounding contraception that can influence adherence to the method.

Efficacy and effectiveness. Effectiveness may be the most important factor of all for many individuals, particularly if a pregnancy would be disastrous. Failure rates are usually given as the percentage of women who experience an unintended pregnancy in the first year of:

- perfect use, i.e. the method is used perfectly but conception occurs
- typical use, i.e. the failure rate when individuals use the method in real life.

Table 1.1 summarizes the effectiveness of currently available contraceptive methods using these criteria.

Contraception needs to be used consistently and correctly for maximum contraceptive benefit. Discussing methods in terms of 'perfect use' is misleading and unfair, when most women will not use a method in this fashion. Methods are often discussed in terms of a spectrum of effectiveness, rather than giving individual percentages. The World Health Organization (WHO) has a simple pictorial chart (Figure 1.2) that compares methods with one another; such a display may have more meaning for a person who is trying to weigh up the difference between 97% and 92% effectiveness. When properly used, the long-acting reversible contraceptives (LARC) – intrauterine devices and systems (IUD/IUS), implants and injectables – offer close to 100% effectiveness. Counseling can help patients weigh up the trade-offs between effectiveness and other factors.

9

TABLE 1.1

Effectiveness of contraceptive methods: percentage of women experiencing an unintended pregnancy during the first year of use and percentage continuing use at the end of the first year

Method	% pregnant		% continuing
	Typical use	Perfect use	
No method	85	85	
Spermicides	29	18	42
Withdrawal	27	4	43
Periodic abstinence	25		51
Calendar		9	
Ovulation method		3	
Symptothermal		2	
Postovulation		1	
Cap, parous women	32	26	46
nulliparous women	16	9	57
Sponge, parous women	32	20	46
nulliparous women	16	9	57
Diaphragm	16	6	57
Condom, female	21	5	49
male	15	2	53
Combined pill and minipill*	8	0.3	68
Combined hormonal patch	8	0.3	68
Combined hormonal ring (NuvaRing)	8	0.3	68
DMPA (Depo-Provera)	3	0.3	56
Copper IUD	0.8	0.6	78
LNG-IUS (Mirena)	0.1	0.1	81
LNG implant (Norplant, Norplant-2)	0.05	0.05	84
Female sterilization	0.5	0.5	100
Male sterilization	0.15	0.1	100

*Combined pills have a lower failure rate than the progestogen-only minipill. DMPA, depot medroxyprogesterone acetate; LNG-IUS, levonorgestrel-releasing intrauterine system.
Adapted from Trussell J. Contraceptive efficacy. In Hatcher RA et al. 2007.

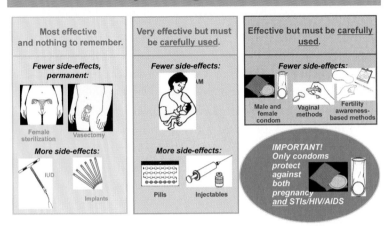

Figure 1.2 WHO decision-making tool for family planning providers
and their clients: comparing methods. Reproduced with permission from
World Health Organization and Johns Hopkins Bloomberg School of Public
Health/Center for Communication Programs © 2005.

Women improve at using a method with practice but, of course,
the cumulative probability of becoming pregnant increases with time,
and no method is 100% effective. The cumulative pregnancy rate (the
probability of getting pregnant over a given period of contraceptive use)
is particularly relevant when considering the efficacy of a long-acting
contraceptive such as the IUD.

Benefits. Highly effective methods clearly reduce the risk of an
unplanned pregnancy, but many methods also have important
and useful non-contraceptive benefits. Highlighting the menstrual
advantages of hormonal contraception, for example, provides extra
motivation to use the method. Women with a strong family history
of cancer could benefit from the risk reduction that prolonged oral
contraceptive use confers. Each method's non-contraceptive advantages
are detailed in the individual chapters.

Providers are often reluctant to discuss contraception with women
who have serious medical conditions, either in the mistaken belief

11

that these women are 'too unwell for contraception' or even too ill to become pregnant. Yet these women often have the greatest need for a safe, effective method.

Risks. 'But what about the risks?' is often asked when discussing contraceptive options. Before getting into the details of the method's risks, it is important to put contraceptive risk in the proper context. For a sexually active woman, the risks of pregnancy are almost always greater than the risks associated with contraception. Women may not have to sign an informed consent to continue a pregnancy, but pregnancy itself carries significant risk (e.g. thromboembolism, pre-eclampsia and hemorrhage). Unintended pregnancy, whether continued or not, also carries profound emotional, social and economic consequences.

All methods of contraception are associated with side effects; some are simply a nuisance while others, albeit extremely rare, may be life-threatening. Some women may choose a less effective but safer method, while others may be prepared to accept higher risks in return for greater efficacy. The importance of individual choice should always be emphasized.

It is not easy to understand the concepts of absolute and relative risk (RR). Many women are concerned about the risks of the combined pill and yet take much greater risks in the course of their lives (Figure 1.3). A 24% increase in the risk of breast cancer (RR 1.24) appears to be a high risk. However, if the absolute risk for a woman of 20 years of age is less than 1 in 10 000 over 5 years, an increase of 24% to 1.24 in 10 000 is a level of risk that most women would accept. People's concerns about risks and side effects may sometimes seem irrational or illogical to professionals who give advice about contraception, but these concerns should be taken seriously as they almost always affect adherence. If a woman's fears remain after discussion, alternative methods should be discussed.

Side effects are among the major reasons for discontinuing contraception. Fear of these problems is also a major reason for not starting certain methods in the first place. Individuals need to know the common side

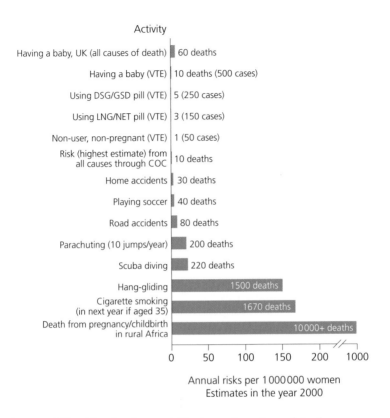

Figure 1.3 provides the data; the following list reflects the chart labels:

Activity

Activity	Deaths
Having a baby, UK (all causes of death)	60 deaths
Having a baby (VTE)	10 deaths (500 cases)
Using DSG/GSD pill (VTE)	5 (250 cases)
Using LNG/NET pill (VTE)	3 (150 cases)
Non-user, non-pregnant (VTE)	1 (50 cases)
Risk (highest estimate) from all causes through COC	10 deaths
Home accidents	30 deaths
Playing soccer	40 deaths
Road accidents	80 deaths
Parachuting (10 jumps/year)	200 deaths
Scuba diving	220 deaths
Hang-gliding	1500 deaths
Cigarette smoking (in next year if aged 35)	1670 deaths
Death from pregnancy/childbirth in rural Africa	10000+ deaths

Annual risks per 1 000 000 women
Estimates in the year 2000

Figure 1.3 The risks of various activities (annual numbers of deaths per 1 000 000 exposed). COC, combined oral contraceptive; DSG/GSD, desogestrel/gestodene; LNG/NET, levonorgestrel/norethisterone; VTE, venous thromboembolism. Reproduced from Guillebaud J. Churchill Livngstone, 2004. With permission from Elsevier, copyright © 2004.

effects of a method and how to tolerate them. Unscheduled bleeding, for example, can be alarming if a woman is unaware it is common when beginning a hormonal method. Many women tolerate irregular bleeding with the subdermal levonorgestrel implant (Implanon) because protection lasts for 3 years, it is extremely effective and the user does not have to remember to do anything. In contrast, the same women may not accept the same bleeding pattern with the progestogen-only pill because of its lower efficacy and the need to remember to take a pill every day. Additionally, certain groups of women – such as athletes or

13

those of particular religious beliefs – may have a low tolerance of unscheduled bleeding.

Women unprepared for a side effect may believe that it is long lasting and dangerous, even if it is temporary and not medically harmful. This is a perfect opportunity for the healthcare professional to dispel myths about a method. Women may have heard worrying rumors from family or friends. They can be reassured that they can always change methods if they are not happy. When individuals discontinue a method on their own, they often do not begin another and are at high risk of unplanned pregnancy.

Use of the method. Never assume that an individual will automatically know how to use the method they have selected; this often applies to condom users as well. Individuals will need brief, well-organized, clear, verbal and written information on how to use their chosen method. They also need information on what to do if a method fails or is used incorrectly (such as with missed pills). Telephone helplines are an extremely valuable way to give back-up information and support. Women not using a LARC method need access to emergency contraception and need to know when and how to use it. The likely challenges to good adherence should be raised: what will she do when she runs out of pills? How will she remember to change her ring? Suggested strategies to improve method use may include marking her patch-change day on her diary/planner or setting a mobile/cell phone alarm to ring daily as a pill reminder.

Other considerations

Contraindications. Although contraception is extremely safe overall, some methods have potentially dangerous (although fortunately rare) consequences. It is very important to elicit any factors in the personal or family history that may increase these risks.

The WHO has published criteria for assessing a woman's medical eligibility for contraceptive use (Table 1.2). The intention is to set international norms for providing contraception to people who have one or more of a range of conditions that may contraindicate one or more contraceptive methods. The document is not meant to provide rigid

TABLE 1.2
WHO medical eligibility criteria for contraceptive use

Category	Classification of condition	Use of the method in practice
1	No restriction for the use of the method	Use in any circumstances
2	The advantages of using the method generally outweigh the theoretical or proven risks	Generally use
3	The theoretical or proven risks usually outweigh the advantages of using the method; requires careful clinical judgment and access to clinical services	Not usually recommended unless other, more appropriate, methods are not available or not acceptable
4	Represents an unacceptable health risk if the contraceptive method is used	Do not use

guidelines, but rather gives recommendations intended to be adapted in line with national health policies, needs and resources. New evidence is incorporated into the guidelines as it becomes available. In the UK, the Faculty of Sexual and Reproductive Health has adapted the WHO's recommendations for the UK population and this UK Medical Eligibility Criteria (UKMEC) reference document is widely used in clinical practice.

Personal and social factors. Multiple other factors need to be considered when choosing a contraceptive method. The list in Table 1.3 may seem extensive, but many questions will be answered in the natural course of taking a clinical history.

STI/HIV prevention. With the rising prevalence of sexually transmitted infections (STIs), including HIV, messages about risk assessment and STI/HIV prevention are now an essential part of the contraceptive

TABLE 1.3

Personal and social factors that affect choice of contraceptive: questions to ask when taking a history

Pregnancy intentions
- Do you want to become pregnant in the near future, years away, or never?

Personal control
- Do you want to be able to stop the method without returning to a healthcare professional?

Privacy
- Is there anyone in your household from whom you are keeping your contraceptive plans a secret?

Partner's intentions and feelings
- Does your partner know you plan on using the method? What are his feelings about contraception?

Presence of medical problems
- Do you have any significant medical problems? (Women with complex medical problems have additional need for highly effective contraception)

Menstrual complaints
- Do you have painful or heavy periods, or other gynecological problems that could benefit from hormonal contraceptives?

Frequency of intercourse
- How often do you have intercourse? (Women who have infrequent intercourse are at a lower risk of pregnancy than women who have intercourse more often, and may make different contraceptive choices)

Method timing
- Do you want a method that you use only at the time of intercourse, or a method that is effective all the time and independent of intercourse?

consultation. Protection against infection is a separate goal from contraception, which individuals may not automatically think about. Both men and women need to know whether the method of contraception that they are relying on protects them against STI/HIV, and that abstinence and the consistent use of condoms are the most effective means of protection available. The use of condoms and another contraceptive – 'dual method' use – provides both STI/HIV protection and greater protection against pregnancy. Individuals need to assess their level of STI/HIV risk, keeping in mind that monogamy may not always be mutual. High-risk individuals may need help with how to negotiate condom use; counseling the couple together or role playing is often helpful.

Key points – choosing a contraceptive method

- Most people use contraception at some stage in their lives and many use it for extremely long periods of time.
- Contraceptive needs change throughout an individual's reproductive life.
- Contraception is essentially safe; it is the *perceived* risk that often deters people from using a method.
- Long-acting reversible contraceptive methods have extremely low failure rates because they make few or no demands on the user.
- Contraceptive users need to balance effectiveness of the method against multiple other factors relating to acceptability. Often, the best contraceptive method is the one the person chooses.
- The World Health Organization publishes a set of regularly updated evidence-based guidelines for safe and effective contraceptive use (www.who.int/reproductive-health/publications/mec).
- Counseling about STI/HIV risk reduction and prevention is an integral part of a comprehensive contraceptive consultation.

Key references

Faculty of Family Planning and Reproductive Health Care. *UK Medical Eligibility Criteria for Contraceptive Use* 2006. www.fsrh.org/admin/uploads/298_UKMEC_200506.pdf

Glasier A, Gebbie AE. *Handbook of Family Planning and Reproductive Healthcare*, 5th edn. Edinburgh: Churchill Livingstone, 2007.

Guillebaud J. *Contraception: Your Questions Answered*, 4th edn. Churchill Livingstone, 2004.

Guillebaud J. *The Pill and Other Forms of Hormonal Contraception: The Facts*, 6th edn. Oxford: Oxford University Press, 2004.

Hatcher RA, Trussell J, Nelson AL et al. *Contraceptive Technology*, 19th edn. New York: Ardent Media, 2007.

Lader D, Hopkins G. Contraception and Sexual Health 2007/08. *Omnibus Survey Report No. 37.* London: Office for National Statistics, 2008. www.statistics.gov.uk/downloads/theme_health/contra2007-8.pdf

Mosher WD, Martinez GM, Chandra A et al. Use of contraception and use of family planning services in the United States: 1982–2002. *Advance Data from Vital and Health Statistics, No. 350.* CDC, 2004. www.cdc.gov/nchs/data/ad/ad350.pdf

National Institute for Health and Clinical Excellence. Long-acting reversible contraception. *Clinical Guideline 30.* London: NICE, 2005. www.nice.org.uk/nicemedia/pdf/cg030niceguideline.pdf

World Health Organization. Comparing effectiveness of family planning methods. Geneva: WHO, 2007. www.fhi.org/nr/shared/enFHI/Resources/EffectivenessChart.pdf [Accessed October 25, 2008].

World Health Organization. Medical Eligibility Criteria for Contraceptive Use, 3rd edn. Geneva: WHO, 2004. www.who.int/reproductive-health/publications/mec/

Introduced in the early 1960s, combined oral contraception (COC) has been used by about 200 million women worldwide. In the USA, more than 18 million women – 30% of women of reproductive age – use COC, and over 80% of women of reproductive age have used COC at some point in their lives. In the UK, there are an estimated 3 million current users and few women over the age of 30 years will have not taken COC at some point.

It is not surprising that the combined pill is so popular; it is extremely effective, easy to use and has multiple health benefits beyond contraception.

The combined pill contains estrogen and a progestogen. Newer delivery systems for combined hormonal contraception (transdermal patch, vaginal ring) have similar contraceptive effects and offer additional choices for women wanting a hormonal method that avoids taking a daily pill. They are particularly useful for the small number of women who experience nausea with the combined pill or who have chronic inflammatory bowel disease, which may be exacerbated by the oral administration of contraceptive steroids.

Oral preparations

Estrogens. COC usually contains ethinyl estradiol and the dose varies from 15 to 50 µg. As the cardiovascular risks of COC are considered to be mainly due to estrogen, preparations containing 50 µg ethinyl estradiol are rarely used and, in the UK, the highest dose preparation remaining on the market is 35 µg. Lowering the dose of estrogen leads to a higher chance of breakthrough bleeding and pregnancy if use is imperfect.

Progestogens. Different progestogens (progestins or synthetic progesterone) have different potencies, and thus contraceptive efficacy is achieved at different doses.

The progestogens used in COC fall broadly into three groups:
- first generation (e.g. norethindrone)
- second generation (e.g. levonorgestrel)
- third generation (e.g. gestodene, desogestrel, norgestimate).

In 2001, Yasmin, a pill containing a new progestogen, drospirenone, was introduced in both Europe and the USA but not Canada. Drospirenone has antiandrogenic and antimineralocorticoid properties, and is said to be associated with a lower incidence of fluid retention and bloating.

Combined oral contraception formulations. Most COC formulations are monophasic preparations in which every hormone pill in the pack contains the same dose of steroids. In biphasic and triphasic preparations, the amounts of both estrogen and progestogen change once or twice during the cycle. There is no evidence for better cycle control with bi- or triphasic pills, and some women find phasic preparations confusing.

The pill has been traditionally taken for 21 days followed by a 7-day break (the pill- or hormone-free interval, PFI or HFI) when withdrawal bleeding usually occurs. Forgetting to restart a packet can allow ovarian follicular growth and ovulation. In the USA, but not in the UK, most women take every-day (ED) preparations in which inactive tablets are taken for the 7 days of the PFI. In theory, ED preparations lessen the chance of lengthening the PFI, thus avoiding the possibility of breakthrough ovulation and risk of pregnancy.

More new formulations of COC are now licensed in which the number of weeks of active pills and the number of days in the PFI vary (Figure 2.1), moving away from the traditional 21/7 model of pill-taking. Their availability varies from country to country.

24/4. Two formulations – YAZ and Loestrin 24 Fe – consist of 24 days of active pills followed by a 4-day PFI/HFI. Both preparations contain 20 µg ethinyl estradiol with different progestogens. These formulations have been shown to have fewer days of bleeding during the PFI and, in theory, they would provide further protection against pregnancy if the start of the next pack was delayed.

84/7. Two formulations in the USA, but not yet in the UK, consist of 84 days of active pills, containing 30 µg ethinyl estradiol and

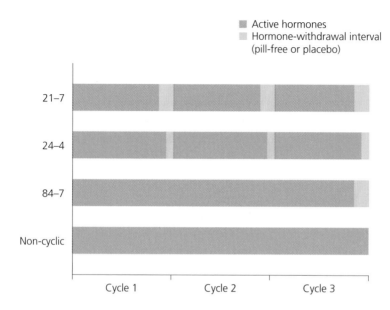

Figure 2.1 Various combined oral contraception formulations.

150 µg levonorgestrel. These are followed by either a 7-day PFI/HFI (Seasonale) or 7 days of tablets containing 10 µg ethinyl estradiol only (Seasonique). These formulations allow for four scheduled bleeding periods per year, though there is an increased chance of unscheduled bleeding or spotting.

365. For years, women using COC have run existing 21-day pill packets together without a break to miss the bleeding episodes. A new product in the USA (Lybrel) can be taken 365 days a year with no placebos at all. Each tablet contains 20 µg ethinyl estradiol and 90 µg levonorgestrel. While 87% of continuing users had no bleeding requiring sanitary protection at 1 year, the remaining users had unpredictable bleeding and spotting episodes.

21/2/5. Another preparation available in the USA, Mircette, consists of 20 µg ethinyl estradiol and 150 µg desogestrel. The active pills are taken for 21 days followed by 2 days of placebo and then 5 days of 10 µg ethinyl estradiol only. This formulation is designed to appeal to women wishing to take the lowest possible dose of estrogen without compromising efficacy or cycle control.

Non-oral preparations

Transdermal contraceptive patch. Evra is a 20 cm^2 matrix patch (latex-free) that delivers a daily dose of norelgestromin, 150 µg, and ethinyl estradiol, 20 µg, into the systemic circulation (Figure 2.2). Each patch is worn for 7 days for 3 consecutive weeks, followed by a patch-free week. Bleeding patterns are not significantly different from those associated with the combined pill, but breast discomfort and dysmenorrhea appear to be slightly more common. It is unclear whether bodyweight affects the patch's efficacy. Several recent studies have suggested an increased risk of venous thromboembolism (VTE) among patch users compared with pill users, while other studies show a similar risk. Women can be counseled that the absolute risk of symptomatic VTE while using the patch is less than the risk of a VTE in pregnancy. Moreover, while VTE has been reported as a potential risk of all hormonal contraceptive therapy (see page 29), it remains a relatively rare event.

Combined contraceptive vaginal ring. NuvaRing is a flexible, soft, transparent ring (latex-free), with an outer diameter of 54 mm and a cross-section of 4 mm, which releases a daily dose of etonogestrel, 120 µg, and ethinyl estradiol, 15 µg, into the vagina (Figure 2.3). The

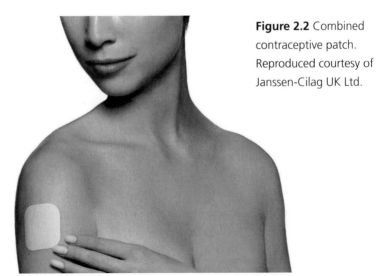

Figure 2.2 Combined contraceptive patch. Reproduced courtesy of Janssen-Cilag UK Ltd.

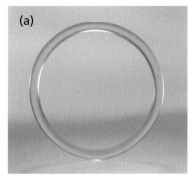
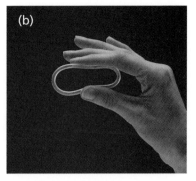

Figure 2.3 (a) Combined contraceptive vaginal ring with an outer diameter of 54 mm and a cross-section of 4 mm. (b) The latex-free ring is soft and transparent, and is easily inserted and removed. Reproduced courtesy of Schering-Plough UK.

ring is worn for 21 days and removed for 7 days, during which time a withdrawal bleed occurs. However, the ring has sufficient hormone for 5 weeks of use and may be worn for more than 21 days. Women may also choose to use successive rings without a break and miss the withdrawal bleed altogether. Cycle control is excellent, with unscheduled bleeding in only 6.4% of cycles. Insertion and removal of the ring is easy; it does not need to fit in any special place in the vagina.

Mechanism of action and effectiveness

Combined hormonal contraception acts mainly by inhibiting ovulation. Estrogen suppresses the development of ovarian follicles, while the progestogen inhibits the development of the luteinizing hormone (LH) surge. Figure 2.4 shows the hormone levels achieved with various delivery systems; Figure 2.5 shows the normal cycle.

Use of combined hormonal contraceptives is also associated with the development of hostile cervical mucus and an atrophic endometrium, so that sperm transport and implantation may be impaired.

When these methods are used perfectly, the failure rate ranges from 0.1% to 2% (1 to 20 pregnancies in 1000 women taking the pill in the first year of use). Typical use, however, is associated with a failure rate of 8%.

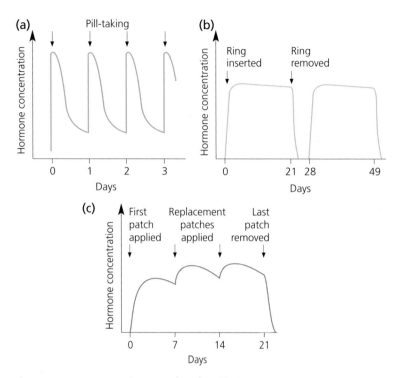

Figure 2.4 Hormone-release profiles for: (a) the oral contraceptive pill; (b) vaginal rings; and (c) patches.

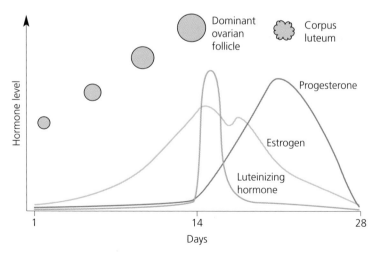

Figure 2.5 Hormone levels and follicle growth in the normal cycle.

Benefits

COC confers a number of non-contraceptive health benefits (Table 2.1). Non-oral preparations are likely to have the same benefits, although there are few specific data available. COC is often the first choice of treatment for menstrual bleeding problems and pain. It is often used to treat acne, and is useful in women with a history of functional ovarian cysts.

COC offers significant protection against both ovarian and endometrial cancer. The combined pill reduces the risk of epithelial ovarian cancer by 20% for every 5 years of use and by about 50% after 15 years of use. Furthermore, some degree of protection persists for 30 years after use has ended. Similarly, the risk of endometrial cancer declines by 40% after 1 year of use and by 80% after 10 years or more. The protective effect lasts for up to 20 years after stopping the pill.

When hormonal contraception is being used for the management of a medical problem the risk–benefit balance changes and the WHO's *Medical Eligibility Criteria* may be less appropriate.

TABLE 2.1

Non-contraceptive benefits of combined hormonal contraception

- Regular and predictable withdrawal bleeding
- Lighter and/or shorter withdrawal bleeding
- Reduced risk of iron-deficiency anemia
- Reduced menstrual pain
- Reduced mid-cycle pain
- Reduced physical premenstrual symptoms
- Reduced cyclic breast pain
- Improved acne
- Reduced risk of functional ovarian cysts
- Reduced risk of ovarian and uterine cancer
- Fewer symptoms of endometriosis
- Reduced risk of pelvic inflammatory disease
- Reduced risk of benign breast disease

Contraindications

Absolute and relative contraindications (category 4 and category 3 conditions in the WHO *Medical Eligibility Criteria*, respectively [see Table 1.2, page 15]) are listed in Tables 2.2 and 2.3, respectively.

Women with hyperprolactinemia wishing to avoid pregnancy should be advised to use progestogen-only contraception; estrogen stimulates

---

TABLE 2.2

Absolute contraindications for use of the combined oral contraceptive pill

- Breastfeeding < 6 weeks postpartum
- Smoking ≥ 15 cigarettes/day and age ≥ 35 years
- Multiple risk factors for cardiovascular disease
- Hypertension: systolic pressure ≥ 160 or diastolic ≥ 100 mmHg
- Hypertension with vascular disease
- Current, or history of, deep-vein thrombosis/pulmonary embolism
- Major surgery with prolonged immobilization
- Known thrombogenic mutations
- Current, or history of, ischemic heart disease
- Current, or history of, stroke
- Complicated valvular heart disease
- Migraine with aura
- Migraine without aura and age ≥ 35 years (continuation)
- Current breast cancer
- Diabetes for ≥ 20 years or with severe vascular disease or with severe nephropathy, retinopathy or neuropathy
- Active viral hepatitis
- Severe cirrhosis
- Benign or malignant liver tumors

Reproduced with permission of WHO *Medical Eligibility Criteria for Contraceptive Use*. 3rd edn. 2004 category 4 conditions (absolute contraindications). Geneva: Reproductive Health and Research, World Health Organization, 2004. www.who.int/reproductive-health/publications/mec/mec.pdf

the lactotrophs, increasing prolactin concentration. Long-term enzyme-inducing drugs, such as some anticonvulsants, griseofulvin or rifampicin (rifampin), may impair the efficacy of the combined hormonal contraceptives, and women on these drugs should consider alternative forms of contraception.

Side effects

Most side effects are minor but often lead to discontinuation. Mood change, weight gain or fluid retention, nausea and vomiting, headache, chloasma, loss of libido, mastalgia and breast enlargement are all quite

TABLE 2.3

Relative contraindications for use of the combined oral contraceptive pill

- Multiple risk factors for arterial disease
- Hypertension: systolic pressure 140–159 or diastolic 90–99 mmHg, or adequately treated to below 140/90 mmHg
- Some known hyperlipidemias
- Diabetes mellitus with vascular disease
- Smoking (< 15 cigarettes/day) and age ≥ 35 years
- Obesity
- Migraine without aura and age ≥ 35 years (continuation)
- Migraine without aura and age < 35 years (initiation)
- Breast cancer with > 5 years without recurrence
- Breastfeeding until 6 months postpartum
- Postpartum and not breastfeeding until 21 days after childbirth
- Current or medically treated gallbladder disease
- History of cholestasis related to combined oral contraceptives
- Mild cirrhosis
- Taking rifampicin (rifampin) or certain anticonvulsants

Reproduced with permission of WHO *Medical Eligibility Criteria for Contraceptive Use*. 3rd edn. 2004 category 3 conditions (relative contraindications). Geneva: Reproductive Health and Research, World Health Organization, 2004. www.who.int/reproductive-health/publications/mec/mec.pdf.

common complaints among pill users, though the evidence to support a causal relationship with the method is inconsistent at best. It is important to let women know that many side effects improve or disappear within 3–6 months of starting the pill, particularly if they are considering changing their method of contraception because of side effects. As some side effects may be alleviated by changing the estrogen dose or type of progestogen, it is worth trying an alternative if time alone does not solve the problem.

Risks

Serious side effects mainly involve the cardiovascular system; the pill affects both venous and arterial circulation. Although the combined pill is associated with alterations in lipids and triglycerides, it is thought that the cardiovascular side effects (both venous and arterial) result from the increased risk of thrombosis.

Myocardial infarction and stroke. The risks of myocardial infarction (MI) and stroke are not affected by the duration of use of COC, and women who have used this form of contraception in the past are not at increased risk for either condition. There is insufficient evidence to prove that the type of progestogen used influences the risk of either stroke or MI.

Myocardial infarction is rare among women of reproductive age. There is almost no increase in the risk of MI among normotensive, non-smoking women who use COC, regardless of age. However, hypertension among pill users increases the risk of MI at least threefold, and diabetes increases the risk by an unknown amount. Smoking greatly increases the risk of MI for women over 35 years of age, and combined methods are therefore contraindicated in this group.

Ischemic stroke is also very rare in women of reproductive age. Among normotensive women who do not smoke, pill use increases the risk of ischemic stroke by about 50% but the absolute risk remains extremely small. The risk is increased by hypertension (threefold) and by smoking (two- to threefold).

Hemorrhagic stroke is not increased in normotensive women under 35 years of age who do not smoke. However, the incidence of hemorrhagic stroke increases with age, and this effect is magnified by use of COC. Hypertension increases the risk by a factor of around 10, and smoking by about 3 times.

Venous thromboembolism (VTE). Current users of COC have an increased risk of VTE 3–6 times that of non-users. The absolute risk is small and much less than that conferred by pregnancy (Table 2.4). The risk probably declines after the first year of use but persists until use of the pill is stopped, when the risk rapidly falls to that of non-users. The risk of VTE is not increased by either smoking or hypertension. Third-generation preparations of COC probably carry a small risk of VTE beyond that of pills containing older progestogens. Given that the absolute risk of VTE remains very small, this differential effect has little impact on clinical prescribing.

Breast cancer. Published studies examining the relationship between COC use and breast cancer have shown inconsistent results. Moreover, their data are difficult to interpret because pill formulations and patterns of reproduction (particularly age at first pregnancy) have changed with time.

In 1996, a large meta-analysis of most of the published data at that time suggested that current or recent use of COC was associated with an increased risk of breast cancer diagnosis. The risk does not seem to be affected by the dose or type of estrogen or progestogen taken, neither is it influenced by the duration of use. After 1 year of pill use, the relative risk of breast cancer increases to 1.24, and it does not rise beyond that figure whether the woman continues to take the pill for 5, 10 or

TABLE 2.4

Incidence of venous thromboembolism per 100 000 women

Never used hormonal contraception	5
Current users: levonorgestrel	15
Current users: desogestrel/gestodene	25–30
Pregnancy	60

20 years. This small increase in risk declines when the pill is stopped; 10 or more years after discontinuing oral contraceptive use, the risk of breast cancer is identical in former users and those who have never used COC. The risk for women with a family history of breast cancer or a personal history of benign breast disease does not appear to be higher than that for women without a personal or family history of the disease.

The exact relationship between the combined pill and breast cancer is still not fully understood. If there is an association, it is possible that pill use results in the earlier detection of tumors or late-stage promotion of the disease.

There is no specific guidance in the UK but the American College of Obstetricians and Gynecologists recommends that a history of benign breast disease or a positive family history of breast cancer (including *BRCA1* or *BRCA2* mutations) should *not* be regarded as contraindications to oral contraceptive use. The *BRCA1* and *BRCA2* mutations are associated with a 45% and 25% lifetime risk, respectively, for epithelial ovarian cancer. Given the reduction in ovarian cancer risk with COC in all women, use of oral contraceptives potentially offers important benefits for women with *BRCA1* or *BRCA2* mutations.

Cervical cancer. Data on the risk of cervical cancer among pill users are also complex and difficult to interpret, as barrier methods confer some protection and the etiology of cervical cancer is linked to sexual activity. Adenocarcinoma of the cervix is rare, but its risk does appear to increase twofold among women using the combined pill. One large study found a fourfold increase in the risk of squamous carcinoma of the cervix among women with persistent human papilloma virus (HPV) infection who have used the pill for more than 10 years. A recent analysis of the same cohort found that long-term use of COC was not associated with increased HPV prevalence. Pill users are a captive population for cervical screening, facilitating early detection and treatment, and almost all squamous carcinoma of the cervix should be preventable in time, as both vaccination and testing for HPV become more widely available (see *Fast Facts: Gynecological Oncology*).

Practical prescribing

A full history should be taken to exclude risk factors that might contraindicate combined hormonal contraception or suggest the need for further investigation.

Blood pressure should be measured, and it may be helpful to record baseline weight.

Pelvic examination is not routinely indicated unless there is reason to suspect gynecological pathology. Women do not like pelvic examinations and most, particularly the young, will be deterred from starting or continuing with the method if examination is seen as a necessary prerequisite. In the *Selected Practice Recommendations for Contraceptive Use*, the WHO recommends that blood pressure measurement is the only test that should be mandatory before starting combined hormonal contraception.

Other routine tests such as cholesterol measurement, are unlikely to contribute substantially to the safe and effective use of the method.

Cervical cytology should be carried out in accordance with national policy. Routine breast examinations are not recommended in the UK or the USA when initiating or continuing hormonal contraception.

Screening for abnormal lipid or coagulation profiles is necessary only for women with risk factors.

Traditional prescribing guidelines suggest starting the method either on the first day of the menstrual cycle, or the Sunday after the start of menses. These guidelines date to a time before sensitive pregnancy testing, and when the effects of hormonal contraception on an early pregnancy were unknown. It is perfectly appropriate to begin a combined hormonal contraceptive method on the day a woman requests it, known as '*Quickstart*'. If a high-sensitivity urinary pregnancy test is negative, a woman can start her pills, patch or ring that day, and should be advised to use a back-up method of contraception (such as condoms) for a week. Bleeding patterns are not greatly disrupted by such initiation of the method. If a woman who has '*Quickstarted*' her contraception does not have withdrawal bleeding by the expected time, she should be instructed to do a pregnancy test.

Use of the method

Women will often say, 'I want a low-dose pill'; all pills in current usage are low dose in comparison with the original preparations. There are no predictors of which hormonal regimen will work for a given woman; a certain degree of trial and error is required. The 'ultra-low-dose' pills (20 µg estrogen) are more likely to lead to breakthrough bleeding.

If women wish to skip the PFI/HFI of their method, they can extend their use of the pill or the ring by immediately beginning another pack at the end of the hormone period. This is not recommended with the patch due to the slightly higher hormone levels.

Other points to remember when prescribing combined hormonal methods are detailed below.

- There is no evidence of any decreased efficacy of these methods while using antibiotics, except when using griseofulvin and rifampicin.
- Women should be carefully instructed about taking COC and what to do when pills are forgotten (Figures 2.6 and 2.7).
- No combined hormonal contraceptive offers protection against HIV infection and other sexually transmitted infections, and this should be made clear to users.
- It is not necessary to take a 'break' from one of these methods, except to try to achieve pregnancy; sustained use of these methods is not harmful. Unplanned pregnancies commonly occur during such breaks – most women who stop taking COC regain their normal fertility within a few months.
- Post-pill amenorrhea can occur but generally lasts less than 3 months. Prolonged amenorrhea is almost always the result of abnormalities present before COC was started, such as polycystic ovary syndrome.
- There is no evidence of any adverse effect on the fetus resulting from previous COC use. If conception occurs during pill use, the risk of teratogenesis is non-existent.

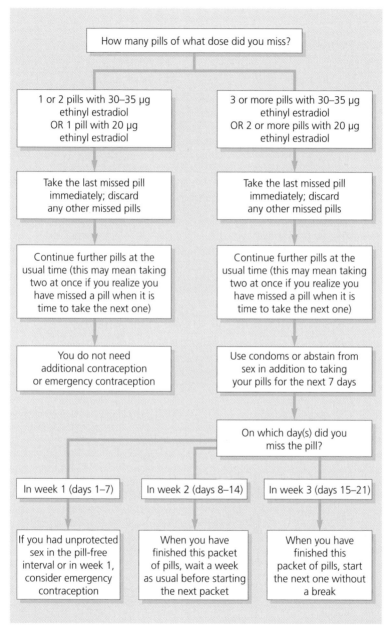

Figure 2.6 Instructions given to women who miss combined pills in the UK.

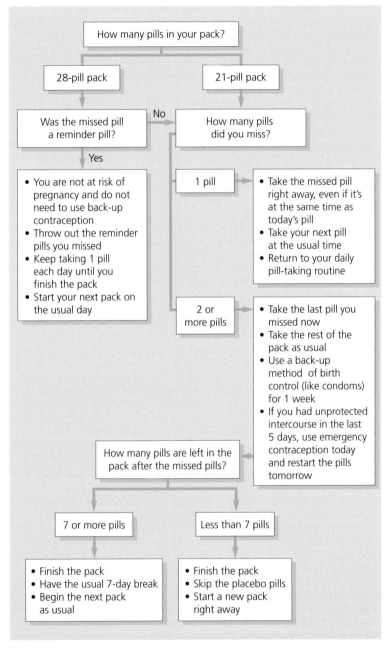

Figure 2.7 Instructions given to women who miss combined pills in the USA.

Key points – combined hormonal contraception

- Combined hormonal contraception is now available via oral (pills), transdermal (patches) and vaginal (rings) routes of administration.
- Failure rates are similar for all methods, at annual rates of around 1 per 100 women with perfect use, and 8 per 100 women with typical use.
- Combined hormonal contraception increases the risk of venous thromboembolism three- to sixfold and slightly increases the risk of stroke, but is not associated with an increased risk of myocardial infarction in non-smoking, normotensive women. The absolute risk of all these conditions is extremely small.
- All combined hormonal contraceptives confer health benefits beyond contraception, particularly in improving menstrual bleeding patterns.
- The pill and the ring can be used continuously to avoid monthly withdrawal bleeds.
- Since these methods require correct and consistent use for optimal efficacy it is important that women are well informed about how to use them.

Key references

ACOG Committee on Practice Bulletins-Gynecology. Use of hormonal contraception in women with coexisting medical conditions. ACOG Practice Bulletin No. 73. *Obstet Gynecol* 2006;107:1453–72.

Beral V, Hermon C, Kay C et al. Mortality associated with oral contraceptive use: 25 year follow up of a cohort of 46 000 women from the Royal College of General Practitioners' oral contraception study. *BMJ* 1999;318:96–100.

Collaborative Group on Hormonal Factors in Breast Cancer. Breast cancer and hormonal contraceptives: a collaborative reanalysis of individual data on 53 297 women with breast cancer and 100 239 women without breast cancer from 54 epidemiological studies. *Lancet* 1996;347:1713–27.

Faculty of Family Planning and Reproductive Health Care Clinical Guidance. First prescription of combined oral contraception. Updated January 2007. www.ffprhc.org.uk/admin/uploads/FirstPrescCombOral ContJan06.pdf

Moreno V, Bosch FX, Muñoz N et al. International Agency for Research on Cancer (IARC) Multicentric Cervical Cancer Study Group. Effect of oral contraceptives on risk of cervical cancer in women with human papillomavirus infection: the IARC multicentric case-control study. *Lancet* 2002;359:1085–92.

O'Connell K, Burkman RT. The transdermal contraceptive patch – an updated review of the literature. *Clin Obstet Gynecol* 2007;50:918–26.

Shimoni N, Westhoff C. Review of the vaginal contraceptive ring (NuvaRing®) *J Fam Plann Reprod Health Care* 2008;34:247–50.

Syrjanen K, Shabalova I, Petrovichev N et al. Oral contraceptives are not an independent risk factor for cervical intraepithelial neoplasia or high-risk human papillomavirus infections. *Anticancer Res* 2006;26: 4729–40.

Vaccarella S, Herrero R, Dai M et al. Reproductive factors, oral contraceptive use, and human papillomavirus infection: pooled analysis of the IARC HPV prevalence surveys. *Cancer Epidemiol Biomarkers Prev* 2006;15:2148–53.

World Health Organization. Cardiovascular disease and steroid hormone contraception. *WHO Technical Report Series No. 877.* Geneva: WHO, 1998.

World Health Organization. Improving access to quality care in family planning. *Selected Practice Recommendations for Contraceptive Use.* 2nd edn. Geneva: Reproductive Health and Research, WHO, 2004. www.who.int/reproductive-health/publications/spr/spr.pdf

Progestogen-only hormonal methods include pills (also known as minipills or POPs), injections, implants and intrauterine delivery systems (the last are covered in Chapter 4). Increasing uptake of long-acting reversible contraceptives (LARC) in the form of implants and injectables is a key strategy in reducing unintended pregnancy in both the UK and USA.

These methods protect against pregnancy by:

- thickening cervical mucus, thus hindering sperm motility
- making the endometrium inhospitable to fertilized eggs
- slowing ovum transport through the fallopian tubes
- suppressing ovulation (depending on the progestogen used and the dose).

Progestogen-only methods can safely be used by almost all women. They are an excellent option if estrogen-containing contraceptives are contraindicated, particularly for women over 35 years of age who smoke, or for women who are at increased risk of thrombosis.

As with combined oral contraception, progestogen-only contraception offers no protection against HIV and other sexually transmitted infections (STIs).

Progestogen-only methods do not reduce breast milk quantity and are a good contraceptive option for lactating women. Progestogens are secreted into breast milk in variable amounts, but no harmful effects on infants have been found.

Progestogen may be less effective if used in combination with drugs that induce liver enzymes, such as barbiturates, rifampicin (rifampin), griseofulvin and St John's wort.

Progestogen-only pills

A small range of pills containing low doses of the older second-generation progestogens (and, in the UK, the third-generation progestogen desogestrel) have failure rates ranging from 0.5% for perfect use to 13% for typical use. If pregnancy does occur while using progestogen-only pills (POPs), the risk of ectopic pregnancy is higher than usual, possibly because progestogens slow ovum transport.

Pill-taking is usually started on the first day of the cycle, but may be started at any point in the cycle ('*Quickstart*', see Chapter 2) with back-up contraception for 7 days. A new packet is begun immediately the day after finishing the previous one; there is no pill-free interval (PFI). The progestogen effect on the cervical mucus peaks within 2–3 hours and then gradually diminishes. The pill must be taken at the same time every day to avoid an increased risk of failure. Women who have missed one or more pills by more than 3 hours should take a pill immediately and then continue taking the pills as usual but also abstain from sex or use additional contraception for the next 48 hours. They should also consider emergency contraception. For women who are breastfeeding and amenorrheic, and are less than 6 months postpartum, no additional contraceptive protection is needed. Breakthrough bleeding is common during POP use, as many women have irregular follicle growth and ovulation and so bleed irregularly.

In the UK, it used to be common practice to advise women weighing more than 70 kg to take two POPs daily. However, with no evidence to support use of double dose POP, this practice is no longer recommended.

POP users return to normal fertility more quickly than women who use combined pills. Side effects such as depression, nausea and breast tenderness also seem less common. Because of disordered follicle growth and ovulation, persistent follicles (with ultrasound appearances of simple ovarian cysts) are common. Most will disappear spontaneously.

A desogestrel-containing pill (Cerazette), 75 µg/day, is available in the UK, but not the USA. This pill differs from older POPs in that the dose of desogestrel inhibits ovulation in almost every cycle of use. In theory, this makes it more effective than the older, lower-dose progestogen-only pills. It also means that the rules for missed pills in this case are the same as for the combined pill (i.e. a 12-hour rule). It has become the POP of choice for young women who for whatever reason cannot take the combined pill.

Depot injection

Depo-Provera is an intramuscular injection of depo-medroxy-progesterone acetate, 150 mg (Figure 3.1). It is widely used in many countries throughout the world.

The contraceptive effect of a Depo-Provera injection lasts for 12 weeks, with a 2-week grace period thereafter, although the manufacturer's licensed use is for up to 12 weeks and 5 days from the previous injection. As with pills, Depo-Provera may be initiated at any point in the cycle if a high-sensitivity urine pregnancy test is negative, and provided a back-up method of contraception (such as condoms) is used for a week (*Quickstart*). The depo-medroxyprogesterone acetate acts as a timed-release depot of progestogen in the muscle. Serum concentration of medroxyprogesterone acetate rises slowly to a peak at about 3 weeks and then gradually decreases until the depot is exhausted. The method is more than 99% effective in the first year of use. Like other progestogen-only contraceptives, Depo-Provera is associated with irregular bleeding, including spotting and long periods of light bleeding. At least 50% of women will have amenorrhea by the end of 1 year of use.

Depo-Provera has a stronger inhibitory effect on ovulation than other progestogen-only methods. As a result, normal fertility does not return as quickly when it is discontinued. The median interval for return of fertility is 10 months – about 6 months longer than those stopping combined oral contraception.

Sickle-cell anemia and seizures may improve on Depo-Provera. The thick cervical mucus resulting from use may offer some protection against pelvic inflammatory disease.

The use of Depo-Provera produces a low estrogen state in women; some studies have shown that this is associated with a loss of bone mineral density (BMD) compared with non-users. However, there is no

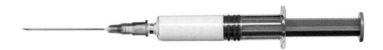

Figure 3.1 Depo-Provera. Reproduced courtesy of Durbin PLC.

evidence that this translates into a higher risk of fracture, and absolute fracture risk is low during the reproductive years. The effect on BMD is largely reversible; relatively few women continue Depo-Provera for long periods. The 2005 World Health Organization Statement on Hormonal Contraception and Bone Health recommends no restrictions on the use of Depo-Provera for women of any age. However, the national regulatory agencies have been concerned about the loss of bone density in adolescents at a time when they would normally be building bone mass. In the UK, the Medicines and Healthcare Regulatory Authority advises limiting the use of Depo-Provera as a first-line contraceptive for adolescents unless other methods are unsuitable or unacceptable; it recommends that all women should be 'reassessed' after using the method for 2 years. This advice tends to be interpreted liberally by clinicians. In the USA, the manufacturer, in consultation with the Food and Drug Administration, has added a warning to its labeling, stating that use of the method for more than 2 years is not recommended unless other contraceptives are found to be 'inadequate'. The American College of Obstetricians and Gynecologists and the Society for Adolescent Medicine, however, have both released policy statements recommending that the use of Depo-Provera should not be limited to 2 years.

Implants

Implanon is widely used in the UK and has become available more recently in the USA. It comprises a single rod that delivers a controlled release of the hormone etonogestrel (3 keto-desogestrel). It is packaged with a disposable inserter for ease of use (Figure 3.2). The implant lasts for 3 years, and the dose of etonogestrel is sufficient to prevent ovulation in all users. The failure rate of Implanon is extremely low and only a tiny number of pregnancies have been reported in women who have had Implanon correctly inserted.

Healthcare providers who insert Implanon need special training. The rod is inserted through a single puncture-type incision of about 3 mm using a trocar. It is usually placed in the inner surface of the upper non-dominant arm and can be easily felt through the skin when positioned correctly (Figure 3.3). The procedure generally takes less than 5 minutes with local anesthesia. Because the incision is so tiny, it seldom leaves a

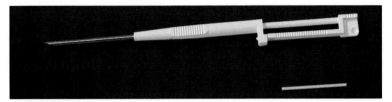

Figure 3.2 The single-rod contraceptive implant Implanon, shown with its disposable inserter.

detectable scar, but inflammation or infection at the insertion site occurs occasionally. If the rod is inserted too deeply, it may be more difficult to remove later. Removal is slightly more difficult than insertion. If the rod cannot be felt, Implanon may be localized with high-frequency ultrasound or MRI.

Implanon should normally be inserted during the first 7 days of the menstrual cycle. If the insertion takes place at any other time during the monthly cycle, use of an additional method of contraception is recommended for the next 7 days.

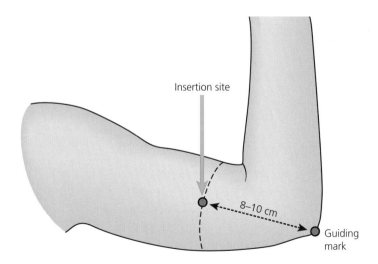

Figure 3.3 Correct location for Implanon placement. The site of insertion is 8–10 cm above the medial epicondyle (arrow). The dotted line shows the insertion point for the needle. Once the needle has been inserted it should be inserted in a line parallel to the humerus.

Irregular bleeding is almost inevitable in users of Implanon and it is impossible to predict the bleeding pattern. Women should be carefully counseled before insertion about change in menstrual bleeding patterns and possible amenorrhea. Prolonged irregular bleeding is the major reason for Implanon discontinuation. Fertility returns almost immediately after the implant is removed.

Norplant comprises six flexible slender silicone capsules that provide a continuous low daily dose of levonorgestrel. The manufacturer recommends 5 years of use. Norplant is virtually as effective as sterilization in the first year of use, with a failure rate lower than 1%; over a full 5-year period, the failure rate is just over 1%. Norplant has now been withdrawn from both the UK and USA, although some women may present to have their capsules removed.

Contraindications

The WHO *Medical Eligibility Criteria* clearly list fewer higher-order contraindications and cautions for progestogen-only pills than for combined pills. Despite this, regulatory agencies in some countries insist that labeled contraindications be the same for progestogen-only and combined pills. In fact, the only category 4 contraindication for all progestogen-only methods (pills, implants and injections) is current breast cancer.

There are several category 3 relative contraindications, which vary according to the specific method and by whether the method is being initiated or continued (Table 3.1).

Those contraindications that apply to injections only are classified as category 3 because of the much higher dose of progestogen in injectable contraceptives.

Risks and side effects

An erratic bleeding pattern is the most notable side effect and is common to all progestogen-only methods. However, total blood loss is usually less than with normal menses. If regular periods are important to a woman, progestogen-only methods may not be a good choice.

TABLE 3.1

Relative contraindications for use of progestogen-only methods

- Breastfeeding < 6 weeks postpartum (all methods)
- Current deep-vein thrombosis or pulmonary embolism (all methods)
- Previous breast cancer with no evidence of disease for 5 years (all methods)
- Active viral hepatitis (all methods)
- Severe decompensated cirrhosis (all methods)
- Benign hepatic adenoma (all methods)
- Malignant hepatoma (all methods)
- Current, or history of, ischemic heart disease or stroke (injections, starting or continuing; continuation of pills or implants)
- Migraine with aura (continuation of all methods)
- Unexplained vaginal bleeding (injections and implants)
- Use of certain drugs: rifampicin (rifampin), griseofulvin, phenytoin, carbamazepine, barbiturates, primidone (pills; implants)
- Multiple risk factors for arterial cardiovascular disease (injections only)
- Hypertension: systolic pressure > 160 or diastolic > 100 mmHg (injections only)
- Vascular disease (injections only)
- Diabetes with nephropathy, other vascular disease or disease duration of > 20 years (injections only)

Reproduced with permission of WHO *Medical Eligibility Criteria for Contraceptive Use*. 3rd edn. Category 3 conditions (relative contraindications). Geneva: Reproductive Health and Research, World Health Organization, 2004. www.who.int/reproductive-health/publications/mec/mec.pdf

It is not unusual for women to report weight gain while using a progestogen-only method of contraception. Fluid retention may also occur, and some women note an increase in the number or intensity of headaches, mood changes, acne or breast tenderness. These reactions may disappear or diminish after several months of use.

Further side effects are noted under the individual formulation types above.

Key points – progestogen-only methods

- Progestogen-only methods are available in many formulations, including pills, injections and subdermal implants.
- Progestogen-only methods probably work by several mechanisms, including suppression of ovulation.
- These methods have few contraindications.
- Classic progestogen-only pills are more likely than combined pills to allow ovulation (and hence pregnancy) if a pill is missed or not taken at the right time.
- A desogestrel-only pill is available in the UK. The dose is sufficient to inhibit ovulation in every cycle, and the missed-pill procedure is the same as for the combined pill.
- Irregular bleeding and amenorrhea are the most notable side effects of progestogen-only methods.

Key references

Croxatto HB. Mechanisms that explain the contraceptive action of progestin implants for women. *Contraception* 2002;65:21–7.

Faculty of Sexual and Reproductive Health. Depo-Provera and young people. Faculty Statement from in the UK. 2004. www.fsrh.org/admin/uploads/Depo_Provera_alert_statement.pdf

Faculty of Sexual and Reproductive Health. Progestogen only implants. Guidance document from the Clinical Effectiveness Unit of the Faculty of Sexual and Reproductive Health in the UK. April 2008. www.fsrh.org/admin/uploads/CEUGuidanceProgestogenOnlyImplantsApril08.pdf

Funk S, Miller MM, Mishell DR et al. Safety and efficacy of Implanon, a single-rod implantable contraceptive containing etonogestrel. *Contraception* 2005;71:319–26.

Mishell DR Jr. Injectable contraception. *J Reprod Med* 2002;47(9 suppl):777–9.

Ortayli N. Users' perspectives on implantable contraceptives for women. *Contraception* 2002;65:107–11.

Porter C, Rees MC. Bleeding problems and progestogen-only contraception. *J Fam Plann Reprod Health Care* 2002;28:178–81.

Westhoff C. Depot-medroxy-progesterone acetate injection (Depo-Provera): a highly effective contraceptive option with proven long-term safety. *Contraception* 2003;68:75–87.

WHO Statement on hormonal contraception and bone health, 2005. Human Reproduction Programme of the World Health Organization. www.who.int/reproductive-health/family_planning/docs/hormonal_contraception_bone_health.pdf

Intrauterine devices (IUDs) are the most commonly used method of reversible contraception worldwide. Nevertheless, they remain the source of more myths and taboos than almost any other method. Intrauterine contraception is growing in popularity in the western world and is highly cost-effective. Healthcare professionals play a key role in giving women balanced information and individual counseling on intrauterine contraception.

Types of intrauterine contraception

The key characteristics of copper IUDs and the Mirena intrauterine system (IUS) are summarized in Table 4.1. Further details of the different types of intrauterine contraception are given below.

Intrauterine devices. IUDs were first introduced in the early 1960s; the original devices were made of plastic. The addition of copper onto the stem of the IUD improved efficacy, allowing the development of smaller T-shaped IUDs with fewer menstrual side effects. The modern 'gold standard' copper devices have more copper wire on the stems than their predecessors, and copper sleeves on the arms, resulting in greater efficacy and a longer duration of action (Figure 4.1).

In the UK, where some 7% of couples using contraception rely on an IUD, seven different copper IUDs are available. They vary in shape, size and in the amount of copper, allowing flexibility of choice to suit the individual woman. In the USA, negative publicity damaged the reputation of the IUD during the 1980s, and nowadays fewer than 2% of American women using contraception use an IUD. Reflecting this decline in popularity, only one copper model (the ParaGard T 380A) is available in the USA.

A frameless IUD is also available in the UK. It comprises six copper beads threaded on to a non-biodegradable polypropylene thread; the top and bottom beads are crimped to keep all the beads in place. The upper end of the thread is knotted and embedded to a depth of 1 cm into the

TABLE 4.1

Key characteristics of copper intrauterine devices versus the Mirena intrauterine system

	Copper IUD	Mirena
Duration of action	Usually 10 years	5 years
Failure rate (first year of use)	0.8%	0.1%
Protection against endometrial cancer	Yes	Yes
Other therapeutic benefits	None	Can use to treat heavy menstrual periods and as part of an HRT regimen
Menstrual spotting	May increase	Increases initially but usually settles within 3–6 months
Hormonal side effects	None	May cause breast pain, fluid retention, acne
Average price	UK £9 $200–400	UK £80 $300–500

HRT, hormone replacement therapy.

fundal myometrium (Figure 4.2). Efficacy appears to be equivalent to the framed copper models, but removals because of pain are fewer.

Intrauterine rings. In China, stainless steel intrauterine rings are still widely used, and immigrant women to the UK and USA may present with these devices. Stainless steel rings cause less menstrual disturbance than modern copper IUDs but are not as effective.

Mirena (intrauterine system). The Mirena, a hormone-releasing intrauterine system (T-frame LNG-20 IUS), has been available for contraception in the UK since 1995. It has a capsule of the progestogen levonorgestrel around its stem from which it releases a daily dose of

47

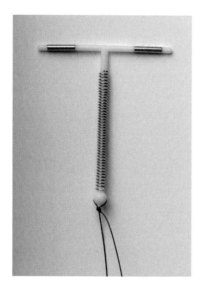

Figure 4.1 Copper intrauterine device with central copper core and copper banding on the arms. Reproduced courtesy of Durbin PLC.

Figure 4.2 The frameless intrauterine device in position. The knot is embedded in the myometrium by means of a special insertion device.

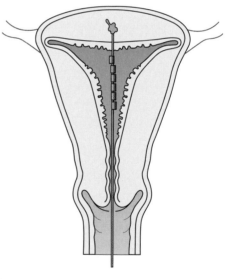

20 μg (Figure 4.3). The only IUS on the market in the UK and the USA, Mirena lasts for 5 years; in the UK, it is also licensed for the treatment of menorrhagia and as the progestogen component of a hormone replacement therapy (HRT) regimen. In the USA, it is not yet licensed for treating menorrhagia but has been approved for contraception since December 2000.

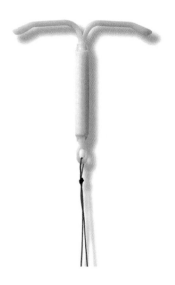

Figure 4.3 The Mirena levonorgestrel-releasing intrauterine system. Reproduced courtesy of Durbin PLC.

Mechanism of action

Copper IUDs stimulate an inflammatory reaction in the endometrium. The concentrations of macrophages, leukocytes, prostaglandins and various enzymes in both uterine and tubal fluid increase significantly. These effects are toxic to both sperm and egg and significantly reduce the chance of fertilization. The effects on the endometrium almost certainly prevent implantation should a fertilized egg reach the uterine cavity.

Mirena induces endometrial atrophy and changes the characteristics of cervical mucus. Ovarian activity is not inhibited, but, as with all low-dose progestogen-only methods, ovarian follicular cysts can persist and are occasionally symptomatic.

Efficacy

The IUD is such an effective method of contraception that it can be justly considered as 'reversible sterilization'. IUDs protect against pregnancy immediately after insertion. Additionally, IUD efficacy rates over years of use are similar to those with tubal occlusion methods. The probabilities of pregnancy during the first year of IUD use and the cumulative pregnancy rates after 7 years of use are shown in Table 4.2.

TABLE 4.2

The efficacy of intrauterine (IUD) contraceptives

	Cumulative pregnancy rate in first year (%)	Cumulative pregnancy rate at 7 years (%)
Copper IUD	0.6	1.7
Mirena	0.1	1.1

Duration of use

Modern copper IUDs last for approximately 10 years, though evidence for some devices suggests efficacy for up to 12 years. Small devices with less copper may only be licensed for 5 years. If a copper IUD is inserted in a woman aged 40 years or older, it can remain in place unchanged until she reaches the menopause. Mirena is licensed for 5 years of use.

Non-contraceptive benefits

Copper IUDs confer a 50–60% reduction in the risk of endometrial adenocarcinoma, possibly due to the intense local inflammatory reaction in addition to complete endometrial shedding every menses.

Mirena. In addition to its high efficacy, Mirena has multiple non-contraceptive benefits (Table 4.3). Most women with Mirena have extremely light periods (about 50%) or amenorrhea (about 20%). After 1 year of use in one study, the average blood loss following insertion of Mirena had decreased by more than 90% among a sample of women with menorrhagia (Figure 4.4). Dysmenorrhea is also reduced. Mirena may also have a therapeutic role for women with endometriosis or small fibroids. When combined with estrogen for HRT, Mirena provides the progestogen necessary for endometrial protection. Estrogen can be given by the woman's preferred route of administration and at a dose titrated against symptom relief.

Contraindications

Women of any age or parity can use intrauterine contraception. While adolescents and nulliparous women have not traditionally been

TABLE 4.3

Non-contraceptive benefits of Mirena

- Reduces total menstrual blood loss in all women
- Reduces blood loss in women with heavy menstrual bleeding (HMB) by over 80%
- Reduces menstrual pain
- Reduces the incidence of fibroids
- May shrink small fibroids
- May reduce symptoms of endometriosis
- May reduce blood loss in women with adenomyosis-related HMB
- May cause regression of endometrial hyperplasia
- Can be used as the progestogen component of hormone replacement therapy

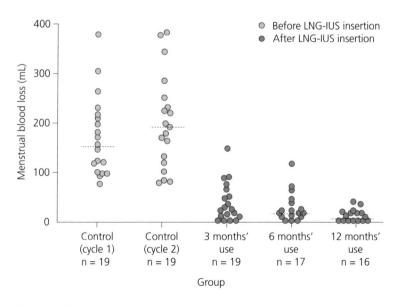

Figure 4.4 Menstrual blood loss among menorrhagic women during two control cycles before insertion of the Mirena (levonorgestrel-releasing intrauterine system; LNG-IUS) and at 3, 6 and 12 months of use. Reproduced with permission from Andersson and Rybo 1990. © Wiley-Blackwell 1990.

considered candidates for an IUD, it should be an option to most of them. The WHO *Medical Eligibility Criteria* give few contraindications to intrauterine contraception. Conditions that are classified as category 4 (an unacceptable health risk) for both copper IUDs and the IUS are listed in Table 4.4.

TABLE 4.4

Absolute contraindications for use of intrauterine contraception

Condition	Category	
	Copper IUD	LNG-IUS
Pregnancy	4	4
Puerperal sepsis	4	4
Immediate postseptic abortion	4	4
Anatomic abnormalities that distort the uterine cavity	4	4
Fibroids that distort the uterine cavity	4	4
Unexplained vaginal bleeding before evaluation	I 4, C 2	I 4, C 2
Malignant gestational trophoblastic disease	4	4
Cervical cancer awaiting treatment	I 4, C 2	I 4, C 2
Current breast cancer	1	4
Endometrial cancer	I 4, C 2	I 4, C 2
Current pelvic inflammatory disease	I 4, C 2	I 4, C 2
Some current STIs	I 4, C 2	I 4, C 2
Known pelvic tuberculosis	I 4, C 3	I 4, C 3

I, initiation; C, continuation; 1, no restriction; 2, advantages outweigh risks; 3, caution, risks usually outweigh advantages; 4, contraindication, unacceptable health risk.
IUD, intrauterine device; LNG-IUS, levonorgestrel-releasing intrauterine system; STI, sexually transmitted infection.
Reproduced with permission of WHO *Medical Eligibility Criteria for Contraceptive Use.* 3rd edn Category 4 conditions (absolute contraindications) Geneva: Reproductive Health and Research, World Health Organization, 2004. www.who.int/reproductive-health/publications/mec/mec.pdf

Side effects

Menstrual disturbance. Copper IUDs cause heavier menstrual bleeding and increased menstrual pain. Bleeding can also be more prolonged and associated with more days of spotting before and after the period. In contrast, the Mirena decreases total blood loss, though many women experience frequent spotting during the first 3 months of use; new users should be advised that this can happen. Women who are well counseled in advance about the method are more likely to tolerate erratic bleeding.

Perforation of the uterus occurs in around 1 of every 1000 insertions and is usually related to the experience of the operator. It is often unnoticed at the time of insertion; a routine follow-up examination 6 weeks after insertion allows most perforations to be detected. Missing threads should be investigated by ultrasound and, if the IUD or Mirena is not seen within the uterine cavity on ultrasound, a plain abdominal X-ray should be taken. At this early stage, a device inside the abdominal cavity can often be retrieved with the laparoscope. If left for months, local adhesion formation around the device often necessitates removal by laparotomy. If the threads have simply been drawn up inside the uterus but the device is in the correct position in the cavity, it can be left in place and the woman reassured that it will be no less effective.

Expulsion rates are around 5% in the first year of use. Expulsion is most common in the first 3 months. Clinicians often advise users to check to feel the IUD threads regularly in order to detect expulsion. In reality, this is often not easy to do and results more often in anxiety than in the detection of unrecognized expulsion.

Ectopic pregnancy. IUDs and the Mirena protect against *all* types of pregnancy, including ectopic pregnancy. However, if pregnancy occurs with an IUD in the uterus, the risk of it being an ectopic pregnancy is around 3–5% (< 1% for Mirena). The risk of an ectopic pregnancy without an IUD in the uterus is approximately 2%. However, as failure is uncommon, the overall risk of ectopic pregnancy with the copper IUD is less than 1.5 per 1000 woman-years of IUD use.

Pelvic infection. The risk of pelvic infection associated with intrauterine contraception has always been overestimated. The IUD does not increase the chance of contracting a sexually transmitted infection (STI), and it does not worsen an infection if one is acquired. The risk of STIs is strongly linked to sexual lifestyle and can be reduced by STI screening for women at increased risk of contracting an infection.

Screening, especially for *Chlamydia*, is recommended before insertion if the woman has any risk factors, i.e. under 25 years of age, recent change of partner, more than one partner in last year etc.

Infection is most likely to occur during the 20 days following insertion. Thereafter, the risk of developing infection is not significantly higher than that among women using no contraception (< 1.5 per 1000 woman-years).

According to the WHO's *Selected Practice Recommendations*, prophylactic broad-spectrum antibiotics are not generally recommended for IUD insertion, but may be considered in settings with a high prevalence of STIs in the local population or limited facilities for STI screening.

If a woman using an IUD is diagnosed with pelvic inflammatory disease, she should be treated with the appropriate antibiotics. The IUD does not need to be removed if she wishes to continue using the method; however, if she does not wish to keep the IUD, it should not be removed until after antibiotics have been started.

Insertion and removal

Intrauterine contraception should be inserted with an aseptic technique. For women who are using effective contraception (including abstinence), an IUD can be inserted at any time in the cycle. Otherwise, insertion should be limited to the first 7 days of the cycle. Postpartum insertion should be within the first 48 hours or delayed until 4 weeks after childbirth, when the risk of expulsion is lower. Particular care should be taken in women who are breastfeeding, as the risk of perforation is higher. An IUD can be inserted immediately after spontaneous or therapeutic abortion, although expulsion rates may be higher after second-trimester abortions.

Unless pregnancy is desired, removal should be undertaken only in the very late luteal phase of the cycle or in the first 7 days. In menopausal women, the IUD should be left for 1 year after the last menstrual period. If the IUD threads are not visible or are pulled off during removal, the device can be removed with a specially designed hook or a pair of artery forceps.

The risk of second-trimester miscarriage, premature delivery and infection are all higher than normal if conception occurs with an IUD in place. If the woman wishes to continue the pregnancy, and if the threads of the IUD are visible (or it can be retrieved safely from the cervical canal), the device should be removed. If removal is not possible it should be left in place. There is no evidence to suggest than an IUD left in situ can cause fetal deformities. If termination of pregnancy is requested, the IUD can be removed at the time of the abortion.

Emergency contraception

The copper IUD (but not the IUS) can be used for emergency contraception (see Chapter 6).

Key points – intrauterine devices and systems

- The intrauterine device (IUD) and Mirena intrauterine system (IUS) both offer extremely safe, long-acting and highly effective contraception.
- The risk of pelvic infection is increased for the first 20 days following IUD or IUS insertion. Thereafter, risk of infection is related to sexual lifestyle.
- The IUD and IUS may be used by women of all ages and parity.
- Intrauterine contraception confers no increased risk of infertility.
- There is a 1 in 1000 risk of perforation and a 1 in 20 risk of expulsion following insertion of intrauterine contraception.

Key references

Andersson JK, Rybo G. Levonorgestrel-releasing intrauterine device in the treatment of menorrhagia. *Br J Obstet Gynaecol* 1990;97:690–4.

Chi I. What we have learned from recent IUD studies: a researcher's perspective. *Contraception* 1993;48:81–108.

ESHRE Capri Workshop Group. Intrauterine devices and intrauterine systems. *Hum Reprod Update* 2008;14:197–208.

Faculty of Sexual and Reproductive Healthcare CEU Guidance document. *Intrauterine contraception.* www.fsrh.org/admin/uploads/ CEUGuidanceIntrauterine ContraceptionNov07.pdf

Grimes DA. Intrauterine devices and infertility: sifting through the evidence. *Lancet* 2001;358:6–7.

Hubacher D. The checkered history and bright future of intrauterine contraception in the United States. *Perspect Sex Reprod Health* 2002; 34:98–103.

IUD Technical Review Committee. IUD Technical Review Committee Meeting Report (Draft). Geneva, Switzerland: World Health Organization, 2006.

Kulier R, O'Brien P, Helmerhorst F et al. Copper containing, framed intra-uterine devices for contraception. *Cochrane Database Syst Rev* 2007;4:CD005347. www.thecochranelibrary.com

Mansour D. Copper IUD and LNG IUS compared with tubal occlusion. *Contraception* 2007;75(6 Suppl): S144–51.

Wildemeersch D. New frameless and framed intrauterine devices and systems – an overview. *Contraception* 2007;75(6 Suppl):S82–92.

Barrier methods of contraception prevent sexually transmitted infections (STIs) and are therefore of enormous importance on a global basis. Condoms are the only contraceptive method that has been shown to prevent infection with human immunodeficiency virus (HIV).

Barrier methods create a physical barrier (condoms, diaphragm, cervical cap) or chemical barrier (spermicide) that blocks sperm from fertilizing an ovum. The male condom is the most commonly used barrier method. Overall, barrier methods are not as popular as hormonal methods but are an important option when presenting the full array of contraceptive choices. They may be used in conjunction with hormonal or intrauterine contraception ('dual-method' use or 'Double Dutch') to increase contraceptive efficacy and personal protection against infection.

Male condoms

Condoms may be made of latex, polyurethane or, rarely in the USA, treated animal tissue. They do not require a prescription, are easily available through many outlets and are often provided free of charge in public health clinics. They are available in differing sizes and shapes; colored, flavored, textured and scented variations are designed to improve their acceptability, particularly to young people.

Condoms are associated with minimal side effects; although some men complain that wearing a condom diminishes pleasure, others find that a small decrease in stimulation allows them to prolong sexual play.

Condoms have a failure rate of 2–15%; couples vary widely in their ability to use condoms consistently and correctly. The difference between 'perfect use' and 'typical use' failure rates is primarily due to incorrect usage – or lack of use – not condom breakage. Healthcare providers may need to teach individuals how to use condoms and can suggest strategies to maximize their effectiveness (Table 5.1; Figure 5.1). Older condoms are more likely to break; only condoms that carry a quality kitemark or similar on the packaging are guaranteed to meet standards.

Emergency contraception is available to prevent pregnancy after condom breakage and slippage (see Chapter 6).

TABLE 5.1

Strategies for maximizing condom effectiveness

ON IN TIME

• Before any genital contact, place the condom on the tip of the erect penis with the rolled side out (see Figure 5.1)

OFF IN TIME

• Immediately after ejaculation, while the penis is still erect, hold the rim of the condom and withdraw the penis

ON EVERY TIME

• Condoms are not effective in their box or on the dresser

NEW ONE EACH TIME

• Use a new condom for each act of intercourse.

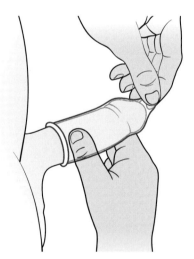

Figure 5.1 Using a condom: leaving approximately 1 cm of space at the top, pinch the top of the condom and roll onto the penis (all the way to the base) with the roll lying on the outside of the condom. Air bubbles can cause the condom to break during sex. Care should be taken not to tear the condom with sharp nails or when removing it from the packet.

Latex condoms are the most widely available and least expensive (less than 50p / $1 per condom). These condoms have been shown to provide very good protection from STIs, including HIV infection. Allergy to latex products or the spermicide that coats some condoms is fairly common. If additional lubrication is desired, it is important to use preparations that will not weaken latex and increase the risk of the condom bursting (Table 5.2).

Polyurethane condoms are more resistant to deterioration but may not protect against STIs as efficiently as latex condoms. Polyurethane transfers body heat readily, so there may be more sensation during sex, and they are compatible with both water-based and oil-based lubricants. These condoms are much more expensive than latex ones but are preferable if either partner has a latex allergy.

'Natural membrane' or lambskin condoms are thinner and stronger than latex, and some men believe they permit more sensation. However, lambskin condoms do not protect against infection, as the membrane's pores, though too small for sperm to pass through, are large enough to allow the passage of microorganisms.

TABLE 5.2

Suitability of lubricants for use with latex condoms

Safe	Not Safe
Egg whites	Baby oil
Saliva	Body or hand lotion
Silicone-based lubricants	Massage oil
Spermicides	Mineral oil
Water	Petroleum jelly
Water-based lubricants	Rubbing alcohol
	Suntan oil and lotions
	Vegetable oils

Female condoms

The female condom is a loose-fitting polyurethane pouch designed to line the vagina. It measures approximately 7.5 cm (3 inches) in diameter and 17 cm (6 inches) in length, lubricated both inside and out (Figure 5.2). The condom has a flexible ring at each end; the slightly smaller ring at the closed end is placed high in the vagina. The ring at the open end remains about 2.5 cm (1 inch) outside the vagina. Like the male condom, each condom should be used once only. Female and male

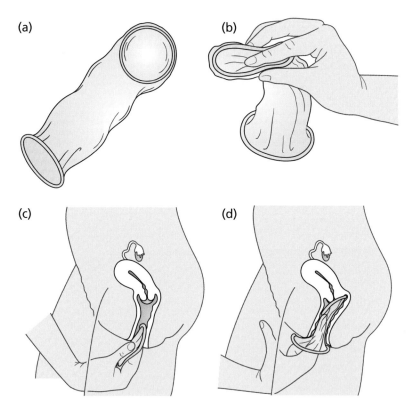

(a) (b) (c) (d)

Figure 5.2 Inserting the female condom: (a) the condom unrolled; (b) the condom in the position for insertion, with the inner ring pinched; (c) the condom is inserted as shown; (d) the inner ring is placed high in the vagina, covering the cervix.

condoms should not be used simultaneously, as they can adhere to each other and cause slippage or displacement.

As the female condom is made from polyurethane, it is less likely to tear or cause allergic reactions than latex. It is not affected by oil-based substances and transfers body heat easily, permitting more sensation. It does not require the use of a spermicide but is compatible with them. Viruses have not been able to penetrate the polyurethane in laboratory tests. The annual rate of pregnancy is listed as 5% for perfect users and 21% for typical users.

Only one version of the female condom is available over the counter in the UK (Femidom) and costs around £1 each. In the USA, the Reality female condom can be bought over the internet and in retail outlets for about $3 per condom.

Spermicide

Spermicide preparations in the USA include foams, gels or creams with applicators, and dissolvable pessaries/suppositories or squares of film. In the UK, the only available spermicide is a single gel preparation. Some spermicidal products are intended to be used with a diaphragm or cervical cap. The active ingredient in all these formulations is nonoxynol-9, which works by damaging the surface membrane of the sperm cell.

Spermicidal products are available over the counter for about £1 / $1–2 per application. They are inserted before intercourse and may require at least a 15-minute wait so they can melt. Most are effective for only 1 hour; another application is needed for a second act of intercourse after more than 1 hour. For typical users, spermicide used alone (without a condom) has a first-year failure rate of 18–29%. There is no association between spermicide use and birth defects.

Spermicide provides some protection against *Chlamydia* and gonorrhea, and possibly against hepatitis B virus infection. Animal studies, however, have shown that the use of nonoxynol-9 facilitates infection with the human papilloma virus (HPV). Nonoxynol-9 kills herpes viruses in vitro, but its in-vivo efficacy has not been demonstrated.

The most common health problem associated with spermicide is irritation of the penis or vagina. This appears to be associated with increased risk of contracting HIV infection among frequent users (multiple times per day) of nonoxynol-9 products. For this reason, it is widely recommended that women at high risk of HIV infection do not use these products for contraception. In addition, use of spermicidal products for lubrication during anal sex is strongly discouraged. Since the addition of nonoxynol-9 to condoms does not increase their effectiveness for contraception or disease prevention, it is recommended that spermicide-coated condoms are no longer used.

Contraceptive sponge

The Today sponge is a small pillow-shaped polyurethane sponge that contains nonoxynol-9 spermicide and has a nylon loop to facilitate removal. It may be placed up to 24 hours before intercourse, and it protects against pregnancy for up to 24 hours no matter how many times intercourse occurs. After intercourse, the sponge should remain in place for at least 6 hours (but not longer than 30 hours as toxic shock syndrome is a concern). Failure rates vary; 'typical use' failure rates are 16% and 32% for nulliparous and multiparous women, respectively. The Today sponge is no longer marketed in the UK. In the USA, it has varying availability, and at the time of this printing was not being manufactured, though remaining stocks were available through the internet.

Diaphragm

The diaphragm is a round rubber hemisphere with a flexible spring rim (Figure 5.3). It is used with a spermicide and fits snugly across the upper vagina, covering the cervix. Diaphragms are available in diameters from 50 to 95 mm; the size needed is related to body size, weight and parity. A trained healthcare professional carries out the fitting, using rings or sample diaphragms. The ideal device is the largest size that is snug without discomfort, touching the walls of the vagina with just enough room to insert a fingertip beneath the pubic bone. The fitting procedure includes a lesson on how to insert and remove the diaphragm. The

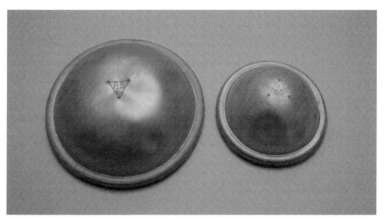

Figure 5.3 Diaphragms.

diaphragm is inserted, with spermicide in the cup, before intercourse, and it should remain in place for 6 hours afterwards (but not longer than 24 hours). Diaphragms can be used during menstruation. They cost about £5–8 / $30–50.

A diaphragm offers some protection against *Chlamydia*, gonorrhea, trichomonas, and possibly HPV. Protection against HIV and other viruses has not been demonstrated.

Some women who wear diaphragms experience repeated urinary tract infections, possibly owing to the pressure of the rim on the urethra and bladder. Diaphragm users or their partners may be allergic to the latex or spermicide.

Failure rates vary from 5 to 21% during the first year. Diaphragms should be examined every few weeks for holes, and the fit should be checked after:

- loss or gain of more than about 9 kg (20 pounds) in weight
- childbirth
- miscarriage
- abortion
- pelvic surgery
- recurring bladder infection.

A diaphragm should also be checked if the user suspects it does not fit.

Cervical cap

The cervical cap is a small latex cup with a firm flexible rim. It is 32–38 mm long (1.25–1.5 inches) and looks like a large rubber thimble. The cap is available in four different inside diameters and fits snugly over the cervix where it is held in place by suction. For a good fit, the inner diameter of the cap must be only 1–2 mm larger than the cervix (Figure 5.4) and the cap should not rest right on the os. About 20% of women cannot get a good fit. Cervical caps cost about £8 / $75.

The cap (plus spermicide) protects against some STIs. It has not been shown to protect against HIV infection. As the cervical cap is latex, it can be damaged by any oil-based substance. It may also irritate the cervix or the penis mechanically or because of latex allergy. It cannot be used during menstruation because it does not permit any flow of secretions.

The cervical cap is used with spermicide placed in its dome. It should be inserted at least 20 minutes before intercourse so that a good seal can develop.

If the cap becomes displaced, women are advised to apply spermicide immediately; emergency contraception should be recommended.

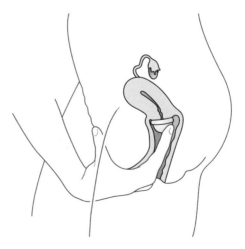

Figure 5.4 Cervical cap, checking placement.

After intercourse, the cap is left in place for at least 6 hours. There is a theoretical risk of toxic shock syndrome if the cap is worn for more than 72 hours, although no cases have been reported.

When the cap is exposed to vaginal secretions it develops an odor, but this can be neutralized by soaking in lemon juice or vinegar solution. Caps usually need to be replaced every 12–18 months. Failure rates range from 8 to 19% during the first year of use.

Lea's shield. A variant of the cervical cap called Lea's shield was approved by the US Food and Drug Administration in March 2002 for use by prescription (Figure 5.5). It is also available over the counter in Canada and parts of Europe but not in the UK.

Because it comes in only one size it does not require fitting. This silicone device is washable and reusable for about a year and has a one-way valve to discharge cervical secretions and air without removal of the cap.

According to its manufacturers, the cap is to be used with spermicide and has a 1-year effectiveness rate of 95%.

The shield should stay in place after intercourse for 6–8 hours but the device should not be left in the vagina for more than 48 hours.

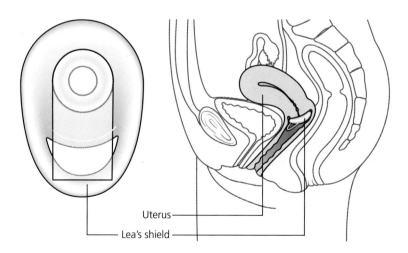

Uterus

Lea's shield

Figure 5.5 Lea's shield and its position.

FemCap. The most recent addition to the array of cervical caps in both the USA and the UK is the FemCap. The device consists of a dome that fits over the cervix, and a flanged brim that extends down along the vagina (Figure 5.6). A strap is attached to the dome for removal.

The FemCap is available by prescription in three sizes (inner rim diameter 22, 26 and 30 mm) – the smallest is intended for women who have never been pregnant, the medium size for women who have been pregnant but have not had a vaginal delivery and the largest size for women who have had a vaginal delivery of a full-term baby.

A groove between the dome and the brim allows placement of spermicide. The device can be worn for up to 48 hours.

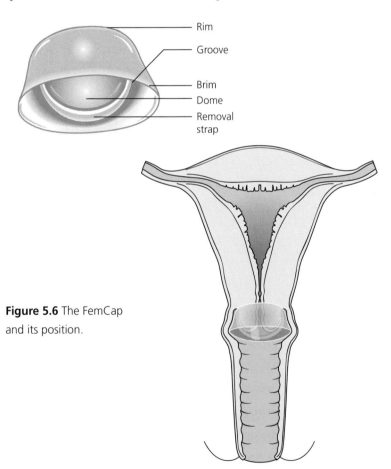

Figure 5.6 The FemCap and its position.

The FemCap is more difficult to insert and remove, and less effective than a standard diaphragm.

Pros and cons

The advantages and disadvantages of barrier methods are shown in Table 5.3.

TABLE 5.3

Advantages and disadvantages of barrier methods

Advantages

- Do not alter hormonal pattern
- Do not cause systemic side effects
- Safe during breastfeeding
- Available over the counter (in most cases)
- Immediate availability no matter how long the interval between uses
- Can be used to bridge a gap before restarting hormonal contraception
- Can be used as a back-up to a fertility awareness method (see Chapter 9)
- Few problems with fit and removal
- Few serious medical problems associated with usage
- Consistent protection against STIs (condoms only)

Disadvantages

- Coital-dependent; intercourse may need to be timed around usage
- Not as effective as hormonal methods or IUDs
- Toxic shock syndrome is potentially life-threatening (but rare)
- Increased risk of skin irritation
- Increased risk of urinary tract infection
- Possibility of latex allergy

IUD, intrauterine device; STI, sexually transmitted infection.

Contraindications

There are virtually no absolute contraindications (category 4 listings) in the WHO's *Medical Eligibility Criteria* for barrier methods. The only cautions (category 3) relate to latex allergy for certain condoms, diaphragms and cervical caps, and for history of toxic shock syndrome for users of the diaphragm and cervical cap.

Key points – barrier methods

- Barrier methods are the only contraceptives that have been shown to protect against sexually transmitted infections.
- All barrier methods require planning and use at the time of intercourse.
- The male condom is the only reversible form of contraceptive for men.
- Spermicides should not be used for contraception by women at high risk of HIV infection or during anal sex.
- With consistent use, barrier methods provide effective contraception.
- Barrier methods present almost no health risks to users.

Key references

Cook L, Nanda K, Grimes D. Diaphragm versus diaphragm with spermicides for contraception. *Cochrane Database Syst Rev* 2003;1:CD002031. www.thecochranelibrary.com

Faculty of Family Planning and Reproductive Health Care. Female barrier methods. Clinical Effectiveness Unit 2007. www.fsrh.org/admin/uploads/ CEUGuidanceFemaleBarrier Methods072007.pdf

Faculty of Family Planning and Reproductive Health Care. Male and female condoms. Clinical Effectiveness Unit 2007. www.fsrh.org/admin/uploads/ 999_CEUguidanceMaleFemale CondomsJan07.pdf

FPA (Family Planning Association). Your guide to diaphragms and caps. London: Sexual Health Direct, 2006. www.fpa.org.uk/attachments/ published/140/PDF%20Diaphragms %20and%20caps%20July%202008. pdf

Gallo MF, Grimes DA, Lopez LM, Schulz KF. Non-latex versus latex male condoms for contraception. *Cochrane Database Syst Rev* 2006;1:CD003550. www.thecochranelibrary.com

Hoffman S, Mantell J, Exner T, Stein Z. The future of the female condom. *Perspect Sex Reprod Health* 2004;36:120–6.

Kuyoh MA, Toroitich-Ruto C, Grimes DA et al. Sponge versus diaphragm for contraception: a Cochrane review. *Contraception* 2003;67:15–18; *Cochrane Database Syst Rev* 2002;3:CD003172. www.thecochranelibrary.com

Mayo Clinic Men's Health. Condoms: STD protection plus effective birth control. www.mayoclinic.com/health/condoms/HQ00463

Minnis AM, Padian NS. Effectiveness of female controlled barrier methods in preventing sexually transmitted infections and HIV: current evidence and future research directions. *Sex Transm Infect* 2005;81:193–200.

Warner L, Steiner MJ. Male condoms. In Hatcher RA, Trussell J, Nelson AL et al. *Contraceptive Technology*, 19th edn. New York: Ardent Media, 2007.

Emergency contraception is defined as any drug or device that is used after intercourse to prevent pregnancy. It is most commonly used after unprotected intercourse or following intercourse in which a condom came off or burst.

Levonorgestrel

Levonorgestrel-only is considered to be more effective than the older Yuzpe regimen (Table 6.1) and as such has become the emergency contraceptive of choice in many countries. It is marketed in the UK as Levonelle and in the USA as Plan B (Figure 6.1). In the UK it can be purchased from pharmacists without a doctor's prescription but is expensive (£25). Some parts of the UK have recently made it available free on the NHS without a prescription, although often restricted to particular age groups such as those under 20 years of age. In the USA, Plan B is now available for purchase directly from a pharmacy without a prescription for women 18 years of age and older. Plan B is still available for adolescents by prescription.

Two dosing regimens are available for levonorgestrel emergency contraception: a single-dose regimen of levonorgestrel, 1.5 mg, taken

TABLE 6.1

Expected pregnancies prevented in relation to the time of administration of emergency contraception

Time (hours) after intercourse	Levonorgestrel (%)	Yuzpe regimen (%)
< 24	95	77
24–48	85	36
48–72	58	31

Adapted from Task Force on Postovulatory Methods of Fertility Regulation 1998.

(a)

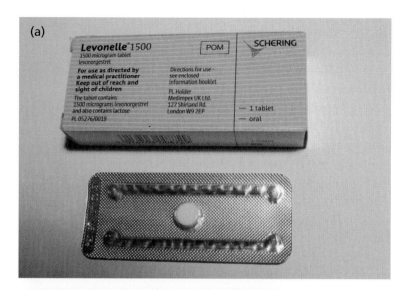

(b)

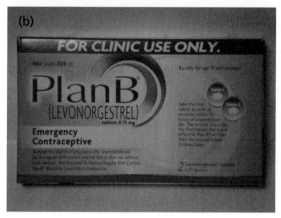

Figure 6.1
Emergency
contraception
available in (a) the
UK – levonelle;
and (b) the USA –
Plan B.

within 72 hours of intercourse is as effective as the older formulation of two 0.75 mg doses 12 hours apart. The single-dose regimen also appears to be effective up to 120 hours after intercourse; it has become the standard formulation in the UK in recent years, and is growing in popularity in the USA. Plan B's current labeling in the USA calls for two doses of 0.75 mg, with the second dose 12 hours after the first.

As levonorgestrel emergency contraception contains no estrogen, side effects such as nausea and vomiting are much less common than with the older hormonal regimens.

71

Yuzpe regimen (combined estrogen–progestogen)

This method, named after the Canadian doctor who first described it, comprises two doses of a combination of ethinyl estradiol, 100 µg, and levonorgestrel, 0.5 mg, given 12 hours apart. There is no longer a dedicated product with this regimen available in either the UK or the USA. It is perfectly possible for women who have combined oral contraceptive pills containing levonorgestrel to make up their own emergency contraceptive. Although few data are available, it seems likely that pills containing other types of progestogen (norethisterone, desogestrel) will work in the same manner.

Copper intrauterine device

The insertion of an intrauterine device (IUD) after intercourse can be used as an alternative to hormonal emergency contraception for up to 5 days after the calculated earliest day of ovulation, or for a single episode of unprotected intercourse at any stage in the cycle.

Modes of action

The mechanism of action of hormonal emergency contraception is not well understood. Both levonorgestrel and the Yuzpe regimen are known to inhibit or delay ovulation, but this is less likely the nearer to ovulation that either drug is given. Taken 5 days before ovulation, both methods will delay or inhibit the process in most women, but taken 2 days before ovulation both methods are much less effective. Both levonorgestrel and the Yuzpe regimen are more effective if they are taken within 24 hours of intercourse than if taken later (see Table 6.1, page 70). For both methods, evidence to support an effect on the endometrium that might inhibit implantation is poor. However, the estimated efficacy of levonorgestrel is greater than can be explained simply by the inhibition of ovulation, so it may act elsewhere in the reproductive process. An alternative explanation is that efficacy has been overestimated, as discussed below.

The copper IUD is known to diminish the viability of ova, as well as the number of sperm reaching the fallopian tube and their ability to fertilize the egg. If it is inserted after fertilization, the IUD works by inhibiting implantation.

Efficacy

This is difficult to calculate for the following reasons.

- Placebo-controlled trials have never been performed and are considered unethical.
- Many users are of unproven fertility.
- The chance of conception with unprotected intercourse in any given cycle is less than 30%.
- It is impossible to know precisely when, in relation to ovulation, treatment has been given (Figure 6.2).

It has become common to describe the efficacy of emergency contraception in terms of the number of potential pregnancies prevented, based on calculating the risk of pregnancy for the day of the cycle on which intercourse occurred. Taken together, accumulated data suggest that levonorgestrel and the Yuzpe regimen prevent 75–85% of expected pregnancies. The IUD is even more effective and probably prevents over 95% of pregnancies.

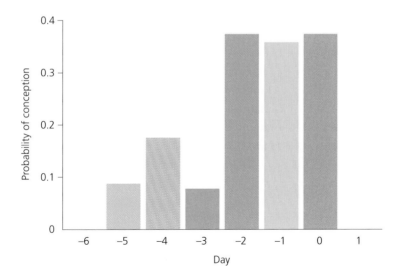

Figure 6.2 The probability of conception occurring after intercourse on the days around ovulation (day 0). Reproduced with permission from Wilcox et al. *N Engl J Med* 1995;333:1517–21. Copyright ©1995 Massachusetts Medical Society. All rights reserved.

Contraindications

There are no absolute contraindications to emergency hormonal contraception. The WHO's *Medical Eligibility Criteria* list several conditions in category 2 (described as 'benefits generally outweigh risks'):

- a history of severe cardiovascular complications (including thromboembolism)
- angina
- migraine
- severe liver disease.

This classification implies that emergency contraception can be provided by someone with limited clinical judgment.

More than one act of intercourse before seeking emergency contraception should not be regarded as a contraindication; it falls into category 1 in the *Medical Eligibility Criteria* ('no restriction for the use of the method'). Emergency hormonal contraception can be given more than once in the same cycle. The user should understand that, if she conceived despite use of the first emergency contraceptive method, a second treatment will not be effective.

There is no evidence that emergency hormonal contraception is teratogenic. However, if there is any possibility that a woman requesting emergency contraception is already pregnant it makes sense to diagnose the pregnancy as this clearly alters the management.

The IUD is not recommended for women at risk of an STI (category 3 – 'the theoretical or proven risks usually outweigh the advantages of using the method'). If there is a risk of infection, the woman should be screened for STIs and the IUD insertion should be covered with broad-spectrum antibiotics.

Side effects

Nausea and vomiting. Around 20% of women taking levonorgestrel alone complain of nausea; after the Yuzpe regimen, up to 60% of women complain of nausea and up to 16% vomit. Many women feel sick with worry, of course. Nausea and vomiting may impact on correct use, particularly if the second dose of the emergency contraception is not taken properly – another reason to encourage a single dose of levonorgestrel when possible.

Breast tenderness. The high dose of estrogen in the Yuzpe regimen may result in breast tenderness for a day or two.

Changes in the next menstrual cycle. Almost 30% of women will experience a delay of more than 3 days in the onset of the next menstrual period. Others will menstruate early. For most women, however, menses will come at the expected time following either hormonal method of emergency contraception.

Difficult/painful IUD insertion may occur, particularly in nulliparous women. Use of local anesthesia should be considered. The risks of infection and perforation are the same as that associated with routine IUD use (see Chapter 4).

Clinical management

Assessment. The date of onset and normality of the last period should be discussed in order to exclude an ongoing pregnancy. To assess the actual risk of pregnancy, the timing of intercourse in relation to the stage of the cycle (see Figure 6.2) and the time elapsed since intercourse should be determined, along with the possible efficacy of the chosen method and the need to consider an IUD. Most of these questions can be answered by the woman using a self-administered questionnaire.

As there are no absolute contraindications to emergency hormonal contraception, blood pressure measurement is not needed. A routine pelvic examination is totally unnecessary and may deter women – particularly young women – from returning for treatment in the future should the need arise. If there is any suspicion that the woman may already be pregnant – for example, if the last menstrual period was abnormal in any way – it is sensible to perform a pregnancy test before prescribing treatment.

Counseling. Women should be informed of current thinking about the way in which emergency contraception acts. They should also be advised of the risk of failure. It is not necessary to ask a woman to sign a consent form before prescribing emergency contraception.

The possible side effects and the effect on the timing of the next menstrual period should be discussed. As the onset of vaginal bleeding is reassuring to women keen to avoid pregnancy, it is important to warn about possible menstrual delay. It should be made clear that emergency contraception does not work by 'bringing on a period'. Women should be advised to have a pregnancy test if the subsequent period does not come or if it is shorter or lighter than usual.

If the need for emergency contraception has arisen as a result of unprotected intercourse, a regular (non-emergency) method of contraception should be discussed and, if appropriate, provided. '*Quickstart*' hormonal contraception, without waiting for the next period, is increasingly being recommended, as many women will be at risk again before their next period. However, as starting hormonal contraception immediately may impair recognition of a delay in menses, some women may prefer to wait and start on the first day of the next menses.

Women should be encouraged to return for emergency contraception should the need arise again. Many women are embarrassed about needing emergency contraception and even more embarrassed about needing it again. Reassure them that taking emergency contraception when they don't wish to become pregnant is a responsible act, and that it is not dangerous to use emergency contraception whenever it is required.

There are some concerns that making emergency contraception available 'off prescription' results in the loss of the opportunity to discuss safe sex and ongoing contraception. Most women do not need to be reminded about these issues; the very fact that they have had to obtain emergency contraception makes many women review their contraceptive practice. As pharmacists extend their role in sexual health, they may be well placed to offer screening for infection in a sensitive manner when women request emergency hormonal contraception.

Improving access to emergency contraception. Women need to recognize when they have to use emergency contraception and need to know how to access it. For example, women requesting condoms can be given information leaflets about using emergency contraception and local availability (Figure 6.3).

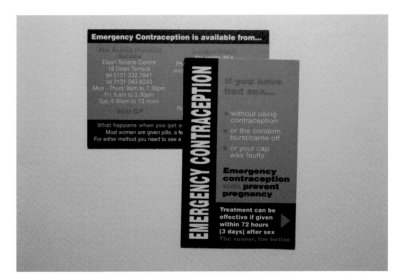

Figure 6.3 An information card about emergency contraception used in Edinburgh, Scotland. It is the size of a credit card, can be kept in a woman's purse and gives information about local availability.

As emergency contraception appears to be more effective if used within 72 hours of intercourse, and may be most effective if used within the first 24 hours, it seems sensible to encourage women to keep a supply at home. One can liken it to bandages – you do not buy them when you cut yourself, you buy them in advance to have on hand when they are needed. In the USA, adolescents can be given prescriptions for Plan B at any visit, so they will always have a valid prescription on hand. A small number of trials of home use in a variety of settings have demonstrated that adolescents and adult women are perfectly able to self-administer emergency contraception and do not tend to abandon more effective contraception in its favor.

Future methods of emergency contraception

Several anti-gestogens have been shown to be effective for emergency contraception. Their efficacy in clinical trials is equivalent, or slightly better, than progestogen-only. None is yet licensed for clinical use in the UK or USA, but one drug is well advanced in its application for this licensed indication in Europe.

Key points – emergency contraception

- Emergency contraception can prevent pregnancy following intercourse.
- Emergency contraception is effective for up to 120 hours after intercourse, but may be more effective the sooner it is taken.
- Available hormonal methods (levonorgestrel and the Yuzpe regimen) appear to work by inhibiting or delaying ovulation.
- Levonorgestrel alone is associated with few side effects, appears to be as effective as the Yuzpe regimen when taken as a single dose (1.5 mg) and is the hormonal method of choice.
- An intrauterine device is a highly effective emergency contraceptive, but insertion requires a trained operator.
- Advanced provision of emergency contraception makes sense and increases use.

Key references

Cheng L, Gülmezoglu AM, Piaggio G et al. Interventions for emergency contraception. *Cochrane Database Syst Rev* 2007;2:CD005497. www.thecochranelibrary.com

Croxatto HB, Devoto L, Durand M et al. Mechanism of action of hormonal preparations used for emergency contraception: a review of the literature. *Contraception* 2001;63:111–21.

Emergency contraception website. Office of Population Research at Princeton University and Association of Reproductive Health Professionals. www.not-2-late.com

Faculty of Family Planning and Reproductive Health Care. Guidance: Emergency contraception. April 2006. www.fsrh.org/admin/uploads/449_EmergencyContraceptionCEU guidance.pdf

Polis CB, Schaffer K, Blanchard K et al. Advance provision of emergency contraception for pregnancy prevention: a meta-analysis. *Obstet Gynecol* 2007;110:1379–88.

Task Force on Postovulatory Methods of Fertility Regulation. Randomised controlled trial of levonorgestrel versus the Yuzpe regimen of combined oral contraceptives for emergency contraception. *Lancet* 1998;352:428–33.

Trussell J, Ellertson C, Dorflinger L. Effectiveness of the Yuzpe regimen of emergency contraception by cycle day of intercourse: implications for mechanism of action. *Contraception* 2003;67:167–71.

von Hertzen H, Piaggio G, Ding J et al. Low dose mifepristone and two regimens of levonorgestrel for emergency contraception: a WHO multicentre randomised trial. *Lancet* 2002;360:1803–10.

Healthy women may remain fertile until their late 40s, yet most have completed their families long before this time. Couples generally choose sterilization for contraception many years before the age of natural sterility in women. In the UK, female sterilization appears to have become less popular over the last decade although the vasectomy rate is stable. The exact reasons for this are complex but women are now often encouraged to use long-acting reversible contraceptive methods and to avoid an operative procedure. Sterilization is the most commonly used contraceptive method in the USA; approximately 700 000 tubal sterilizations and 500 000 vasectomies are performed annually.

Female sterilization involves a surgical procedure to obstruct or bisect the fallopian tubes, thus preventing sperm from reaching an egg. Sterilization surgery is performed most often on an outpatient or day-case basis, with procedures that usually take less than 30 minutes. Surgery has no effect on hormone production, ovulation, menstruation or sexual function.

Techniques
Female sterilization is most often performed by laparoscopy or mini-laparotomy. The type of surgery depends on:
- timing of the procedure
- the health of the woman
- the preferences of the surgeon
- the hospital or clinic facilities
- the woman's preference for type of procedure, incision or anesthesia.

Alternatively, the fallopian tubes can be blocked by microinserts placed via hysteroscopy into the fallopian tubes (Essure).

Mini-laparotomy. If sterilization is performed immediately after childbirth, a mini-laparotomy is preferred, because this approach is easiest when the uterus and tubes are high in the abdomen. An incision of approximately 3 cm is made below the umbilicus, allowing access to each tube.

Overweight women and those with adhesions from previous surgery may need a laparotomy for interval tubal ligation (4–6 weeks postpartum). An incision of approximately 5 cm is made low in the abdomen, often just above the pubic hair, for both access and cosmetic reasons. The incision is closed with sutures or staples.

Laparoscopy is the most common approach to female sterilization in the UK and USA. It is extremely safe when performed by an experienced surgeon. It is often done as an outpatient procedure, which reduces cost.

Various methods are used to block the fallopian tubes (Figure 7.1). A high-frequency electric current may be applied briefly to the narrow middle section of the fallopian tube (electrocoagulation). Scars then develop and block the tube permanently. The tubes can also be blocked by pinching them shut with mechanical devices such as metal clips (Filshie clips) or small silastic rings (Fallope rings) that are like strong

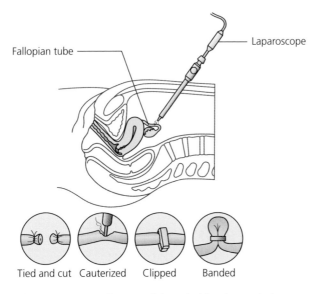

Figure 7.1 Laparoscopy and some of the tubal ligation techniques commonly used.

rubber bands. Eventually the pinched tissue necroses, forming a permanent seal. Alternatively, sutures can be used to tie each tube, after which the surgeon removes the section of the tube between the ties. The procedure costs approximately £800–£1000 / US$2500–5000.

Anesthesia. Laparoscopic sterilization or mini-laparotomy can be done under local anesthesia because these short procedures cause little trauma to the tissues. General anesthesia or epidural and spinal blocks, however, are routinely used in both the UK and USA.

Essure, a new non-surgical system for female sterilization, is available in both the UK and USA. Trained providers use a hysteroscope to guide insertion of a small metal coil (Figure 7.2) into each fallopian tube using a thin catheter (Figure 7.3). The outpatient procedure requires no, or only local, anesthesia. The Dacron mesh embedded in the coils causes scar tissue to grow and block the tubes. This process takes 3 months to complete and, in that interval, women must use another means of contraception. At 3 months, imaging must be performed to confirm bilateral tubal occlusion. In the USA, the manufacturers recommend a hysterosalpingogram. In the UK, pelvic radiography is usually the first step, although ultrasound and contrast infusion sonography are further techniques that can be used to confirm adequate microinsert location.

For women relying on Essure for contraception after successful placement of the device, an effectiveness rate of 99.74% after 5 years of follow-up has been reported. The procedure is cheaper than laparoscopic sterilization and costs somewhere in the range of £700 / US$1500–2500.

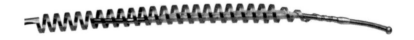

Figure 7.2 Essure micro-insert.

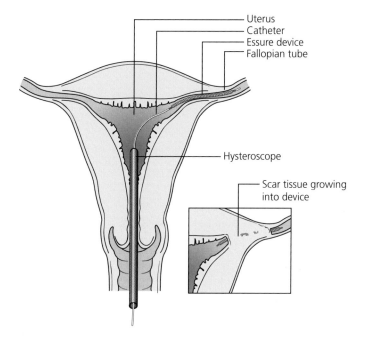

Figure 7.3 Insertion and action of the Essure device.

Effectiveness

Female sterilization is one of the most effective contraceptive methods, with a failure rate of 0.2–2% over a 10-year period. Efficacy is somewhat dependent on the procedure; rare pregnancies have been reported with Essure, while sterilization via bipolar cautery has the highest failure rate of the modern methods. The greatest risk of failure occurs in younger women, who tend to be more sexually active and more fertile. Occasionally, failure occurs because an occluding device did not work properly or because electrocoagulation was not complete. In addition, a channel can re-form in an incompletely sealed tube, allowing eggs or sperm to pass through.

Reversibility

Women should never have a tubal occlusion if there is a chance that some day they might want to have it reversed. It is possible to repair occluded fallopian tubes so that they can function again, but success rates vary widely (20–70%). Success of tubal reversal depends on two factors:

- the type of tubal ligation procedure originally performed
- the age of the woman at the time she seeks tubal ligation reversal.

With regard to the type of procedure originally performed, sterilization procedures that destroy too much of the tube or remove the fimbria make reversal impossible, and electrocoagulation causes extensive destruction. A procedure that uses a clip or silastic band has the greatest chance of reversal. Women over 40 are likely to have decreased fertility due to age, in addition to the tubal factors.

Nothing is yet known about the reversibility of the Essure procedure, but it is likely to be technically extremely difficult.

Benefits

Female sterilization is ideal for women who are certain that their childbearing is complete. It is a highly effective, safe, permanent method of contraception, with privacy of choice and no need for partner compliance. Once done, it relieves women of the hassle of future contraception choice. There are no absolute medical contraindications to female sterilization. Evidence also consistently shows that sterilization is associated with a reduced incidence of ovarian cancer and pelvic inflammatory disease.

Risks and possible complications

The WHO's *Medical Eligibility Criteria* for female surgical sterilization deal mostly with the risks associated with surgery and general anesthesia (where used). Delay is advised when women have acute transient conditions that may make surgery more dangerous (e.g. pneumonia, sexually transmitted infections [STIs], eclampsia). Caution is necessary when women are suffering from chronic problems that make surgery or anesthesia more dangerous (e.g. cardiac disease, diabetes, hepatic cirrhosis). There are no criteria for the Essure procedure, since the guidelines were developed before that system became available.

Deaths resulting from female sterilization surgery are extremely rare (1–4 in 100 000); they arise mostly from complications from the use of general anesthesia. Major complications – including injuries that require further surgery to repair – occur in 1–2 of every 1000 laparoscopy patients. The risk of complications from laparoscopy is influenced considerably by the skills of the surgeon. Clinicians who perform sterilization require special training and sustained experience is important. Surgeons who carry out fewer than 100 laparoscopies each year tend to have a much higher rate of complications.

Pregnancy. Because the risk of pregnancy after sterilization is uncommon, the overall risk of ectopic (tubal) pregnancy is lower among these women than in the general population. However, roughly 30% of post-sterilization pregnancies are ectopic. Women who undergo sterilization should be carefully counseled that if they ever miss a menses or have physical signs of pregnancy they should do a pregnancy test and seek early evaluation.

Regret. Due to the permanence of the procedure, careful counseling is important before sterilization. The risk of regret overall is about 10–15%. This risk, however, is higher among women under the age of 30 (about 20%), who may be more likely to experience life changes, and women who undergo sterilization within a year of delivery (about 21–23%). Other risk factors for regret include having received less information about other contraceptive options, less information about the procedure, and making the decision under pressure from their family or spouse.

Counseling
Several factors should be discussed when counseling a woman, and preferably her partner, about female sterilization.
- Long-acting reversible contraceptive methods have comparable efficacy but are reversible.
- Sterilization is a permanent procedure (there is no 5- or 10-year tubal).
- Sterilization is not perfect. Many women are surprised to hear that pregnancy is possible after tubal occlusion.
- There is a risk of ectopic pregnancy, should a pregnancy occur.

- The chance of regret may be higher if a woman has recently given birth.
- Sterilization does not protect against STIs; thus, unless in a mutually monogamous relationship, couples still need a barrier method, preferably condoms.
- Sterilization does not remove the need for regular gynecological care, including cervical cytology tests.
- Women choosing sterilization do not need to be married but the possibility of partnership change is an important factor when considering sterilization as a contraceptive method.
- Although partner consent is not required, it is a good idea for a woman to include her partner in the decision-making process, when possible.

Key points – female sterilization

- Female sterilization is an extremely effective, safe and well-accepted way to prevent pregnancy.
- There are many techniques for female sterilization, all of them best performed by a surgeon with special training.
- Most sterilizations can be carried out using local or regional anesthesia and without hospitalization.
- A non-surgical method of female sterilization (Essure) is also available.
- The timing of sterilization should be up to each woman after she has carefully considered her situation, including the wishes of her partner if she chooses to involve him.
- Sterilization should be considered permanent, because reversal, although technically possible, is costly, involves major surgery and is often not successful.

Key references

Curtis KM, Mohllajee AP, Peterson HB. Regret following female sterilization at a young age: a systematic review. *Contraception* 2006;73:205–10.

Kulier R, Boulvain M, Walker D et al. Minilaparotomy and endoscopic techniques for tubal sterilisation. *Cochrane Database Syst Rev* 2004;3:CD001328. www.thecochranelibrary.com

National Institute for Clinical Excellence (NICE). Hysteroscopic sterilisation by tubal cannulation and placement of intrafallopian implants. *Interventional Procedure Guidance 44.* February 2004. www.nice.org.uk/nicemedia/pdf/ip/IPG044guidance.pdf

Peterson HB. Sterilization. *Obstet Gynecol* 2008;111:189–203.

Pollack AE, Thomas LF, Barone MA. Female and male sterilization. In Hatcher RA, Trussell J, Nelson AL et al. *Contraceptive Technology,* 19th edn. New York: Ardent Media, 2007.

Royal College of Obstetricians and Gynaecologists (RCOG). Male and female sterilisation. *National Evidence-Based Clinical Guidelines No. 4.* 2nd edn. London: RCOG, 2004.

Sagili H, Divers M. Hysteroscopic sterilisation with Essure: a promising new alternative to tubal ligation? *J Fam Plann Reprod Health Care* 2008;34:99–102.

Vasectomy, the sterilization procedure for men, is simpler and safer than female sterilization and is usually performed in an outpatient setting. A vasectomy takes only a few minutes to perform, is almost 100% effective, has few complications and is permanent. In the UK, slightly more men than women now choose sterilization, whereas in the USA, the ratio of men to women sterilized is 1:2.5.

In a vasectomy, the two sperm ducts (vas deferens) that carry sperm from the testicles to the penis are cut. A small portion of each vas is removed, and the cut ends are closed off. A vasectomy does not influence virility, nor does it have any negative impact on overall health. The only change that takes place is that the semen contains no sperm, so it cannot cause pregnancy. A man can remain fertile for 2–4 months after the procedure, until all the sperm that were present when the surgery was performed have been ejaculated (up to 20 ejaculations) or have died. Another contraceptive method should be used until two consecutive specimens of semen are found to be free of sperm.

A vasectomy does not protect either partner against sexually transmitted infections.

Techniques

The standard vasectomy technique uses a tiny incision (Figure 8.1); the 'no-scalpel' method uses a puncture (Figure 8.2). Some incisions are so small that they need no suture. Very small forceps are used to pull the vas up through the incision or puncture. To sever the vas deferens, the surgeon may:

- cut and tie, removing a short portion of tissue
- use clips
- use electrocautery to seal the ends of the vas deferens.

All of these techniques seem to produce equally good results.

Sperm will still be produced by the testicles and may build up behind the closed end of the vas. The accumulation can sometimes be painful.

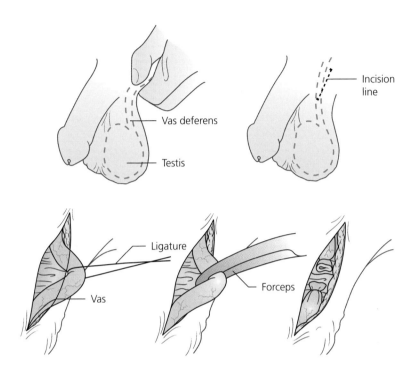

Figure 8.1 The standard vasectomy technique.

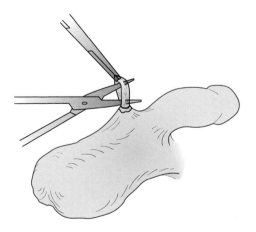

Figure 8.2 The 'no-scalpel' vasectomy.

Fortunately, sperm have a short lifespan; they soon die off and are absorbed by the body. Some surgeons may leave open one end of the vas deferens, closing only the section that connects with the penis. This allows sperm to spill and not accumulate in the delicate epididymis. Although a vasectomy that closes off only one end may be more easily reversible, it also has a greater chance of failure.

The 'no-scalpel' method, developed in China in the 1970s, is associated with a greatly reduced risk of hemorrhage. The approach takes only about 10 minutes and causes considerably less soreness, bleeding and bruising afterwards.

Most vasectomies take about 20 minutes. After a brief recovery period at the clinic, men are advised to rest at home for 24 hours to allow the incision to heal. Men who do physical labor are generally advised to wait for 1 week before going back to strenuous work. All men who have had vasectomies should wear an athletic support or jockey shorts for 4–6 weeks to support the scrotum until it is completely healed. The rule for having intercourse after a vasectomy is to wait until it feels comfortable, anywhere from a few days to 2 weeks.

Efficacy

Vasectomy is highly effective and should not be considered reversible. Although it is possible to repair the occluded vas, this requires delicate microsurgery, which is not always successful.

A typical first-year failure rate for vasectomy is 0.5–1.0%. Pregnancies can result from:

- unprotected intercourse before the reproductive tract has been totally emptied of the sperm present when the surgery was performed
- a closed vas reconnecting
- accidental interruption of a structure other than the vas deferens in the sterilization procedure, leaving the vas intact.

Reversibility

Like tubal occlusions for women, vasectomies can sometimes be reversed successfully. As the diameter of the inner canal of the vas deferens is approximately that of a pinpoint, a surgeon must use a microscope when rejoining the ends of these almost invisible tubes.

Because this requires major surgery, it is done under general anesthesia, is expensive and requires a long recovery time. Patency of the tube may be established, but pregnancy may still not occur because of the development of antisperm antibodies. Pregnancy rates following a reversal procedure vary from 16 to 79%, with the majority of clinics achieving a success rate close to 50%.

Because successful reversal is difficult, the decision to opt for male sterilization should be given long, careful thought and be accompanied by good counseling. Before undergoing this operation, it is essential for a man to feel comfortable with the fact that a vasectomy is permanent. Partner consent is not required, but it is a good idea for a man to include his partner in the decision-making process if possible.

Contraindications

There are very few contraindications to vasectomy listed in the WHO's *Medical Eligibility Criteria*. If there is local skin infection, systemic infection or gastroenteritis, filariasis or an intrascrotal mass, the WHO tables recommend delaying the vasectomy until the problem has resolved or been investigated. Caution is recommended in the presence of a large varicocele or hydrocele, cryptorchidism or previous scrotal injury (any of which may make surgery technically more difficult), or if the man is diabetic (since wound healing may be compromised). Vasectomy should be undertaken in an appropriately specialized unit if the man has AIDS or a coagulation disorder, or requires a simultaneous hernia repair.

Complications

Complications after vasectomy occur in only a fraction of procedures. They include:

- hematoma (1.6%)
- infection (1.5–3.4%)
- epididymitis (1.4%)
- sperm granulomas (0.3%).

Sperm granulomas (nodules caused by the presence of sperm that have leaked from one end of the severed vas) need surgery only if they are painful.

Side effects

Although an association between vasectomy and prostate and testicular cancer has been suggested, there is no good evidence to substantiate this and no biologically plausible reason for an association.

Hormonal male contraception

Over the last decade, major effort has gone into the attempted development of hormonal regimens for male contraception. Studies have found that spermatogenesis can be inhibited by progestogens, antiandrogens and gonadotropin-releasing hormone analogs. However, these treatments can interfere with sexual function, necessitating add-back therapy with testosterone to maintain libido and erectile function. Testosterone can only be given by a non-oral route for this role; testosterone therapy also increases the risks of both cardiovascular and prostate disease. Research is ongoing but at the present time the prospect of a safe and effective male hormonal method remains an elusive concept that is unlikely to be available in the near future.

Key points – vasectomy and hormonal methods for men

- Vasectomy is highly effective and the procedure is simple.
- A variety of techniques for interrupting the vas deferens exist; they appear to be equally effective.
- 'No-scalpel' vasectomy is associated with less bleeding and pain than other methods.
- No good evidence substantiates the suggested association between vasectomy and prostate and testicular cancer.
- Although fertility can be restored after vasectomy, success rates are low.
- A safe and effective method of hormonal male contraception has not yet been developed, although research is ongoing.

Key references

Cook LA, Pun A, van Vliet H et al. Scalpel versus no-scalpel incision for vasectomy. *Cochrane Database Syst Rev* 2007;2:CD004112. www.thecochranelibrary.com

Cook LA, van Vliet H, Lopez LM et al. Vasectomy occlusion techniques for male sterilization. *Cochrane Database Syst Rev* 2007;2: CD003991. www.thecochranelibrary.com

Holt SK, Salinas CA, Stanford JL. Vasectomy and the risk of prostate cancer. *J Urol* 2008;180:2565–7.

Jamieson DJ, Costello C, Trussell J et al. The risk of pregnancy after vasectomy. *Obstet Gynecol* 2004; 103:848–50.

Peterson HB. Sterilization. *Obstet Gynecol* 2008;111:189–203.

Royal College of Obstetricians and Gynaecologists (RCOG). Male and female sterilisation. *National Evidence-Based Clinical Guidelines No. 4*. 2nd edn. London: RCOG, 2004.

Schuman LM, Coulson AH, Mandel JS et al. Health status of American men – a study of post-vasectomy sequelae. *J Clin Epidemiol* 1993;46:697–958.

Wenk M, Nieschlag E. Male contraception: a realistic option? *Eur J Contracept Reprod Health Care* 2006;11:69–80.

Fertility-awareness-based (FAB) methods are based on identifying the 'fertile window' – the only time when fertilization is likely during the menstrual cycle. Although menstrual cycles vary in length, the 'fertile phase' is almost always the same length. Some methods involve tracking cycle days to determine which days a woman is most likely to be fertile. Other methods involve observing and interpreting the body's signs of fertility.

Successful use of FAB methods depends on learning which days are fertile and either refraining from penetrative intercourse or using another form of contraception on those days. An abstinence approach can mean avoiding penetrative sex for one-third to one-half of the month.

Traditional fertility-observation methods have no negative physical side effects and the costs are low to the user. However, to be successful these methods require serious commitment and diligent practice. Table 9.1 summarizes the most common FAB methods.

Physiological basis

Early in the cycle, the pituitary releases follicle-stimulating hormone, which stimulates a number of follicles in the ovary to grow and secrete estrogen. This causes the cervix to produce more mucus. The cervical os widens as the mucus becomes abundant, watery and 'stretchy'. The increased level of estrogen also stimulates the pituitary to secrete luteinizing hormone (LH). The resulting surge of LH triggers the release of a mature ovum from its follicle, which then begins to produce progesterone. Stimulation by this hormone causes changes in both the quality and the quantity of cervical mucus, and increases the basal body temperature (BBT).

Temperature remains measurably elevated until progesterone level declines. When the progesterone concentration falls, the endometrium begins to be sloughed off, menstruation occurs and the cycle begins

TABLE 9.1

A summary of fertility-awareness-based methods of contraception

Method	Observations per cycle	Days of abstinence
Standard Days	Track cycle days beginning with day 1 of menses	12 days
Calendar/rhythm	Identify shortest and longest cycles among preceding 6–12 cycles	Depends on cycle length variability
TwoDay	Presence or absence of cervical secretions	Approximately 10–14 days
Billings ovulation	Daily cervical secretions	Approximately 14–17 days
Temperature	Daily basal body temperature	Approximately 17 days
Symptothermal	Daily secretions and basal body temperature	Approximately 12–17 days

again (see Figure 2.5, page 24). Ovulation occurs approximately 14 days before the onset of menstruation, regardless of the total length of a woman's menstrual cycle.

Ova are viable for only 12–24 hours, but sperm can survive in the reproductive tract for as long as 7 days. Ovulation predictor kits, available in pharmacies and drug stores to help women conceive, can detect ovulation 24–48 hours beforehand by detecting the LH surge (e.g. Clearblue/Clearblue Easy with urine and Ovacue with saliva). Given sperm's survival ability, this is not soon enough to alert a couple to avoid intercourse. In the UK, a computerized monitor (Persona) is available, which takes readings of urinary hormone levels and predicts safe (green light) and unsafe (red light) days for contraceptive purposes. The monitor reads red on 6–10 days a month, indicating the need for a barrier method or abstinence to avoid pregnancy.

Efficacy

The effectiveness of FAB methods is dependent on three factors:
- the ability of the method to predict the fertile days in the cycle
- the ability of the woman/couple to identify these fertile days
- the ability of the woman/couple to abstain from intercourse or use a back-up method during these fertile days.

FAB methods work best for highly motivated older couples that have used them consistently. Among perfect users, first-year failure rates vary from 1 to 5%. Among typical users, however, 10–25% become pregnant during the first year.

Standard Days method

This method is most appropriate for women who usually have cycles between 26 and 32 days long. The first day of menstrual bleeding is considered day 1. The couple may have unprotected intercourse from days 1 to 7. Intercourse should be avoided, or a back-up method used, from days 8 to 19. The couple may have unprotected intercourse again from day 20 to the end of the cycle. Many women who use the Standard Days method use a color-coded string of beads called CycleBeads to help them keep track of their cycle days (Figure 9.1).

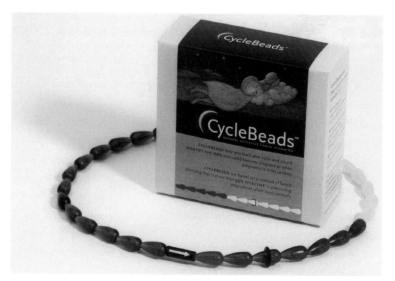

Figure 9.1 CycleBeads. Reproduced courtesy of Cycle Technologies Inc.

Calendar/rhythm method

On a calendar of 6 to 12 menstrual cycles, fertile days are calculated by subtracting 18 from the length of the shortest cycle and 11 from the length of the longest cycle. These two numbers represent the beginning and the end of the fertile days for the current cycle (Table 9.2). The woman should update the calculation every cycle to determine the fertile days for each cycle.

TwoDay method

The TwoDay method is based on the presence or absence of cervical secretions. A woman checks for secretions every day, in the afternoon and evening, by looking at the secretions on her underwear or toilet

TABLE 9.2

Fertile day calculation with the calendar/rhythm method

If your shortest cycle length is...	Then the first day of the fertile period is...	If your longest cycle length is...	Then the last day of the fertile period is...
20 days	Day 2	25 days	Day 14
21 days	Day 3	26 days	Day 15
22 days	Day 4	27 days	Day 16
23 days	Day 5	28 days	Day 17
24 days	Day 6	29 days	Day 18
25 days	Day 7	30 days	Day 19
26 days	Day 8	31 days	Day 20
27 days	Day 9	32 days	Day 21
28 days	Day 10	33 days	Day 22
29 days	Day 11	34 days	Day 23
30 days	Day 12	35 days	Day 24
31 days	Day 13	36 days	Day 25
32 days	Day 14	37 days	Day 26
33 days	Day 15	38 days	Day 27

paper, touching the secretions on her vulva and feeling the sensation of wetness on her vulva. If she noticed any secretions *today* or *yesterday*, she can become pregnant today. If she did not notice any secretions today or yesterday she is not fertile today.

Billings ovulation method

Changes in mucus can signal the onset of the fertile period. The cervical glands secrete very little mucus immediately after menstruation. After a few 'dry' days, the mucus remains scant, but becomes sticky and appears somewhat white, yellow or cloudy. When this type of mucus is present, unprotected intercourse is no longer safe. Women should be advised that semen can be confused with mucus, so secretions on a day following intercourse should be considered with caution.

A few days before ovulation, the mucus becomes much more abundant, clear, slippery and very 'stretchy'. The last day on which this type of mucus occurs is the day of peak fertility. Peak fertility has only definitely passed when the mucus becomes sticky and scant again (3–4 days after the peak fertility day). Women are not fertile from this time until after menstruation and when the fertile phase of the next cycle begins. Vaginal infections, douching or any use of lubricant or spermicidal jelly will make it difficult to interpret mucus changes.

Temperature method

BBT, or resting temperature, is charted for 3 or 4 months to establish fertility patterns. After ovulation, the BBT usually rises by between 0.22 and 0.44°C (0.4 and 0.8°F) and remains at that level until just before the start of menstruation (Figure 9.2). A woman can safely consider herself to be not fertile after 3 days of raised temperature. BBT is taken in the morning before rising and before eating or drinking. It can be measured orally, rectally or vaginally, but the same method should be used every time. Because the temperature rise is triggered by progesterone after ovulation, this method cannot be used to warn of ovulation. Illness, travel, alcohol consumption and a later rising time can raise the BBT; given the amount of potentially confounding cofactors, the temperature method is best used in conjunction with another method.

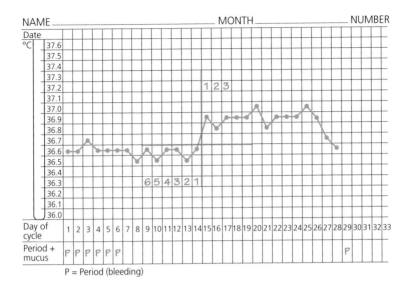

NAME _____ MONTH _____ NUMBER

Figure 9.2 Basal body temperature chart demonstrating the acute rise due to ovulation. Reproduced with permission from Glasier and Gebbie *Handbook of Family Planning and Reproductive Healthcare*. 5th edn. Churchill Livingstone © Elsevier 2008.

Symptothermal method

This combines checking cervical mucus, recording BBT and watching for the other signs of ovulation. For example, during the infertile phase the cervix is lower in the vagina, easier to reach and firm to the touch. As ovulation approaches, the cervix becomes higher, broader and softer. Cervical secretions can help identify the start of the fertile phase.

After ovulation, the cervix is again low in the vagina and feels firm and closed. The infertile period begins:

- after 3 days of increased BBT
- after 3 days of a closed, firm, low cervix
- 4 days after the peak fertility day.

This combined approach is particularly useful for women with unusually short or long cycles.

Advantages

FAB methods are relatively inexpensive (more expensive if electronic daily monitoring is used), have no side effects and do not require a prescription or a visit to a healthcare provider. These methods may be the only ones acceptable among women of particular religious faiths. Knowledge of the signs of fertility can help a woman become pregnant when she is ready, and to help detect impaired fertility.

Disadvantages

FAB methods, like all non-barrier methods, provide no protection against sexually transmitted infections. The male partner's cooperation is essential for successful use and may be difficult to obtain consistently.

Contraindications

FAB methods lack efficacy in certain situations and cannot be recommended at these times (Table 9.3). Particular FAB methods are not recommended for women:

- with irregular cycles (Standard Days)
- unable to correctly interpret signs of fertility (Billings ovulation, Symptothermal)
- unable to recognize the presence of secretions (TwoDay)
- with a vaginal infection that increases secretions (TwoDay).

TABLE 9.3

Times at which fertility-awareness-based methods are not recommended

- Recent childbirth
- Current breastfeeding
- Recent menarche
- Recent discontinuation of hormonal contraceptive methods
- Intermenstrual bleeding not distinguishable from menstruation or that mask normal secretions
- Perimenopause

Key points – biologically based methods

- A woman's monthly hormonal cycle produces observable clues to her fertility.
- Couples can use knowledge of female physiology to avoid pregnancy.
- Biologically based methods are heavily dependent on individual behavior for effectiveness.
- Methods based on periodic abstinence tend to have high failure rates when used typically.

Key references

Frank-Herrmann P, Heil J, Gnoth C et al. The effectiveness of a fertility awareness based method to avoid pregnancy in relation to a couple's sexual behaviour during the fertile time: a prospective longitudinal study. *Hum Reprod* 2007;22:1310–9.

Freundl G, Godehardt E, Kern PA et al. Estimated maximum failure rates of cycle monitors using daily conception probabilities in the menstrual cycle. *Hum Reprod* 2003;18:2628–33.

Jennings VH, Arevalo M. Fertility awareness-based methods. In *Contraceptive Technology*, 19th edn. Eds Hatcher RA, Trussell J, Nelson AL. New York: Ardent Media, 2007.

Trussell J, Measuring the contraceptive efficacy of Persona. *Contraception* 2001;63:77–9.

The last thing on the average woman's mind after she gives birth is 'When can I do this again?' The postpartum period of infertility may be unexpectedly brief and very dependent on the frequency and duration of any breastfeeding. In a time of healing incisions and sleep deprivation, many women will not be thinking about contraception when they leave hospital. Accordingly, counseling about postpartum contraception ideally should take place prenatally.

Clinicians often have worries about prescribing contraception in the postpartum period because of concerns regarding both maternal and neonatal health. However, the very small theoretical risks of the method must be weighed up against the very real risks for some women of early conception. While many women will attend their standard 6-week postpartum check-up, some will not. Many women will become sexually active before this visit, further emphasizing the need for a contraceptive plan before hospital discharge.

During pregnancy, cyclic ovarian function is suppressed. Estrogen and progesterone produced by the placenta support the pregnancy, as well as inhibit the pulsatile pituitary release of follicle-stimulating hormone (FSH) and luteinizing hormone (LH). Postpartum, FSH and LH levels gradually rise in response to the decreased levels of estrogen and progestogen.

Most non-lactating women will resume menses within 4–6 weeks of delivery, although many cycles are anovulatory – up to 85% of cycles in the first 6 months.

The timings of when to initiate postpartum contraception are summarized in Table 10.1.

In breastfeeding women

Lactational amenorrhea method. Breastfeeding extends the period of infertility and depressed ovarian function due to disruption of the

TABLE 10.1

When to initiate postpartum contraception

Timing after delivery	Breastfeeding women	Non-breastfeeding women
Immediately	• Tubal occlusion • LAM • Copper IUD (within 48 hours) • Condoms and spermicides • Withdrawal	• Tubal occlusion • Copper IUD (within 48 hours) • Progestogen-only methods • Condoms and spermicides • Withdrawal
3 weeks	• Progestogen-only implant • Progestogen-only pills	• Combined E/P methods
4 weeks	• Mirena • Copper IUD	• Mirena • Copper IUD
6 weeks	• Tubal occlusion • DMPA • Combined E/P methods* • Diaphragm and cervical cap	• Tubal occlusion • Diaphragm and cervical cap
6 months	• Combined E/P methods	
Any time	• Abstinence • Vasectomy	• Abstinence • Vasectomy

*Check national guidelines.
DMPA, depot medroxyprogesterone acetate; E/P, estrogen/progestogen;
IUD, intrauterine device; LAM, lactational amenorrhea method.

pulsation of gonadotropin-releasing hormone (Figure 10.1). In the right circumstances, using breastfeeding as the sole means of contraception – the lactational amenorrhea method (LAM) – is more than 98% effective (Figure 10.2).

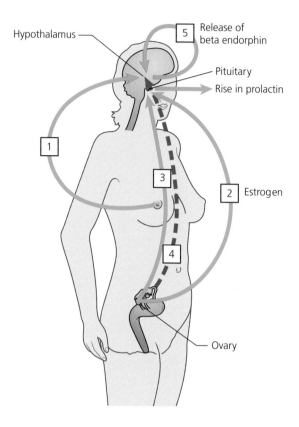

Figure 10.1 Possible mechanisms of lactational amenorrhea. Nerve impulses from the nipple produce:

- a rise in the level of prolactin produced by the pituitary (1)
- changed hypothalamic sensitivity to ovarian steroid feedback (2)
- altered gonadotropin secretion (3).

Whether prolactin contributes directly to the changes in hypothalamic sensitivity or blocks gonadotropin activity at the level of the ovary is not established (4). Suckling may also stimulate the release of beta endorphin, which suppresses gonadotropin-releasing hormone from the hypothalamus (5). Adapted from *Contraception During Breastfeeding: A Clinician's Sourcebook*. 2nd edn. New York: Population Council, 1997.

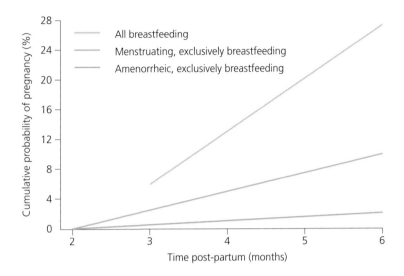

Figure 10.2 Cumulative probability of pregnancy in breastfeeding women. Reproduced from *Contraception During Breastfeeding: A Clinician's Sourcebook*. 2nd edn. New York: Population Council, 1997.

When LAM works. Women who use LAM successfully must be:
- amenorrheic – no return of bleeding at all
- exclusively breastfeeding
- within 6 months of postpartum – even if the other criteria are met.

When LAM doesn't work. LAM is unsuccessful under the following circumstances:
- menses have returned, even if irregular
- frequency of feeds has been reduced
- duration of time between feeds has increased
- night feeding has stopped, or the infant is sleeping through the night
- bottle feeding or regular food supplements have been introduced
- pumping or hand-expressing milk for all feeds is not as effective as suckling for contraception.

Women who breastfeed beyond 6 months postpartum or after the return of menses can combine breastfeeding with other contraceptive methods for enhanced effectiveness.

Hormonal methods. There are concerns about using hormonal contraception during lactation, although they are not supported by evidence. Because falling progesterone levels trigger lactogenesis, early initiation of hormonal contraceptives could theoretically interfere with this process. Combined estrogen–progestogen contraceptives are thought to suppress milk production in the early postpartum period. Contraceptive hormones will be excreted in very small amounts into breast milk (< 1% of the maternal dose). However, the levels of hormones in breast milk when using a hormonal method of contraception is comparable to levels observed when women have an ovulatory cycle. Finally, the immature metabolism of neonates theoretically could lead to accumulation of hormones and their metabolites in the infant.

A systematic review of randomized clinical trials investigated the effects of hormonal contraception (progestogen-only pills, combined estrogen–progestogen pills, injectables) on the volume of breast milk, the initiation, maintenance and duration of breastfeeding, and infant growth. The review found:

- insufficient evidence to establish if hormonal contraception has any effect on breast milk quantity or quality
- hormonal contraception does not have an adverse effect on infant growth or development.

Progestogen-only. If hormonal methods are to be used, progestogen-only contraceptives (pills, injectables, implants, Mirena) are the preferred method for breastfeeding women, although timing of initiation of therapy is somewhat controversial. Manufacturers recommend starting progestogen-containing oral contraceptives 6 weeks postpartum if the mother is exclusively breastfeeding, and 3 weeks postpartum if she is supplementing with formula. However, no data are available on the impact of earlier initiation of progestogen-only contraception. According to manufacturers' guidelines, the Mirena intrauterine system (IUS) may be inserted 6 weeks postpartum.

The World Health Organization (WHO) states that the risks of progestogen-only methods for breastfeeding women outweigh the benefits in the first 6 weeks postpartum (category 3). Contrary to manufacturers' guidelines (see above), the WHO supports insertion of the Mirena from 4 weeks postpartum, regardless of the method of infant feeding.

The American College of Obstetricians and Gynecologists (ACOG) recommends that breastfeeding women initiate progestogen-only oral contraceptives at 2–3 weeks postpartum, and depot medroxy-progesterone acetate (DMPA) at 6 weeks postpartum. In certain clinical situations, such as concern about patient follow-up, ACOG states that it may be appropriate to start progestogen-containing contraception earlier.

The Faculty of Sexual and Reproductive Health Care (FSRH) in the UK adapted the WHO's *Selected Practice Recommendations* as a whole, but no consensus was achieved on a recommendation for the initiation of progestogen-only pills and implants. A subsequent FSRH guidance document recommends that breastfeeding women initiate the progestogen-only pill at 3 weeks postpartum, progestogen-only implants between 3 and 6 weeks, and DMPA at 6 weeks postpartum. In situations where a breastfeeding woman is at risk of pregnancy and is unwilling to consider alternative methods, implants may be considered before 3 weeks, and DMPA may be considered between 3 and 6 weeks postpartum. Like the WHO, the FSRH supports insertion of the Mirena from 4 weeks postpartum.

Combined estrogen–progestogen. Expert recommendations on the initiation of combined methods in breastfeeding women vary.

The WHO recommends delaying the initiation of combined contraceptives until 6 months postpartum (Category 4 in the first 6 weeks postpartum). Between 6 weeks and 6 months, the WHO states that the theoretical or proven risks usually outweigh the advantages of the method (Category 3).

ACOG recommends delaying the initiation of combined estrogen–progestogen contraceptives until at least 6 weeks postpartum, and then only if breastfeeding is well established and the infant's nutritional status can be closely monitored.

The FSRH in the UK does not recommend the use of combined methods before 6 weeks postpartum in breastfeeding women, but advises that they can be used without restriction from 6 months. It states that breastfeeding women should be informed that the combined pill is not recommended between 6 weeks and 6 months postpartum but, if breastfeeding is established, they may be considered if other contraceptive methods are unacceptable.

Non-hormonal methods

Intrauterine device. Breastfeeding women can safely use a copper intrauterine device (IUD), as the device has no effects on breast milk. The IUD may be inserted:

- immediately after the expulsion of the placenta (immediate postpartum insertion)
- within 48 hours of delivery (delayed postpartum insertion)
- 4 weeks postpartum because of the increased risk of perforation (interval insertion).

IUD insertion should be delayed when there has been premature rupture of membranes or after prolonged labor or fever because of elevated risk of infection. The IUD can be inserted immediately after a Cesarean delivery through the hysterotomy incision. Expulsion rates are higher for postpartum insertion (6–10%) than for those following interval insertion, but are lower for immediate insertion than for delayed postpartum insertion.

Barrier methods. The use of condoms and spermicides may begin immediately postpartum. The use of diaphragms and caps should be postponed until involution of the uterus is complete (about 6 weeks postpartum), at which time the device can be properly (re)fitted. There is an increased risk of toxic shock syndrome when lochia is present.

Non-breastfeeding women

Hormonal methods

Progestogen-only contraceptives (pill, injection, implant) may be safely initiated immediately postpartum and should be initiated by 2 weeks after delivery.

Combined estrogen–progestogen methods (pill, patch, ring) may be initiated 3 weeks after delivery; this delay is due to the risk of postpartum thromboembolism. Since a woman may not return for a check-up before 4–6 weeks postpartum, she should be given a prescription for her method when she leaves the hospital.

Mirena (intrauterine system). As for breastfeeding women, the Mirena IUS may be inserted 6 weeks postpartum according to the manufacturer's guidelines. The WHO and FSRH, however, support insertion of the Mirena from 4 weeks postpartum.

Non-hormonal methods
Tubal occlusion may be performed after vaginal delivery or at the time of Cesarean delivery.

Copper IUD. Insertion guidelines are the same as those for breastfeeding women – insertion may take place immediately after placental delivery or at the time of Cesarean delivery, within 48 hours of delivery or postponed until 4 weeks postpartum.

Barrier methods. As with breastfeeding women, the use of condoms and spermicides may begin immediately postpartum. The use of diaphragms and caps should be postponed until involution of the uterus is complete (about 6 weeks postpartum), at which time the device can be properly (re)fitted. There is an increased risk of toxic shock syndrome when lochia is present.

Key points – postpartum contraception

- Exclusive breastfeeding is a highly effective form of contraception for up to 6 months postpartum.
- Exact timings of initiation of hormonal methods in breastfeeding women vary according to national guidelines.
- Clinical considerations, such as a woman's pregnancy risk and refusal to use other contraceptives, may impact when a clinician chooses to initiate hormonal contraception in the postpartum period.

Key references

Faculty of Family Planning and Reproductive Health Care. Contraceptive choices for breastfeeding women. *J Fam Plann Reprod Health Care* 2004; 30:181–9.

Faculty of Family Planning and Reproductive Health Care. *UK Selected Practice Recommendations for Contraceptive Use* developed through a FFPRHC expert consensus meeting 2002. Adapted from WHO *Selected Practice Recommendations for Contraceptive Use* 2002. www.fsrh.org/admin/uploads/breastfeeding.pdf

Kennedy KI, Trussell J. Postpartum contraception and lactation. In *Contraceptive Technology*, 19th edn. Eds Hatcher RA, Trussell J, Nelson AL. New York: Ardent Media, 2007.

Truitt ST, Fraser AB, Grimes DA et al. Combined hormonal versus nonhormonal versus progestin-only contraception in lactation. *Cochrane Database Syst Rev* 2003;2:CD003988. www.thecochranelibrary.com

Truitt ST, Fraser AB, Grimes DA et al. Hormonal contraception during lactation. Systematic review of randomized controlled trials. *Contraception* 2003;68:233–8.

Useful resources

UK
Faculty of Sexual and
Reproductive Healthcare
of the Royal College of
Obstetricians and Gynaecologists
27 Sussex Place, Regent's Park
London NW1 4RG
www.ffprhc.org.uk

fpa
(formerly Family Planning
Association)
50 Featherstone Street
London EC1Y 8QU
Tel: +44 (0)20 7608 5240
www.fpa.org.uk

Medicines and Healthcare products Regulatory Authority
10–2 Market Towers
1 Nine Elms Lane
London SW8 5NQ
Tel: +44 (0)20 7084 2000
info@mhra.gsi.gov.uk
www.mhra.gov.uk

USA
American College of
Obstetricians and Gynecologists
409 12th St, SW, PO Box 96920
Washington, DC 20090-6920
Tel: +1 202 638 5577
www.acog.org

Association of Reproductive Health Professionals
1901 l Street, NW, Suite 300
Washington, DC 20036
Tel: +1 202 466 3825
www.arhp.org

Contraception Online
Baylor College of Medicine
Houston, Texas
www.contraceptiononline.org

The Guttmacher Institute
125 Maiden Lane, 7th Floor
New York, NY 10038
Tel: +1 212 248 1111
Toll-free: 1 800 355 0244
www.guttmacher.org

US Food and Drug Administration
5600 Fishers Lane
Rockville, MD 20857-0001
www.fda.gov

International
Geneva Foundation for Medical Education and Research
Chemin Edouard-Tavan 5
1206 Geneva, Switzerland
Tel: +41 (0)22 346 7716
info@gfmer.org
www.gfmer.ch

Population Council
One Dag Hammarskjold Plaza
New York, NY 10017, USA
Tel: +1 212 339 0500
pubinfo@popcouncil.org
www.popcouncil.org

World Health Organization
Avenue Appia 20
1211 Geneva 27, Switzerland
Tel: +41 22 791 2111
info@who.int
www.who.int
Reproductive health resources:
www.who.int/reproductivehealth/
publications/index.htm
WHO *Medical Eligibility Criteria
for Contraceptive Use*, 3rd edn,
2004:
www.who.int/reproductive-
health/publications/mec/
WHO *Selected Practice
Recommendations for
Contraceptive Use*, 2nd edn, 2004:
www.who.int/reproductive-
health/publications/spr/

Index

What the reviewers say:

"This concise, up-to-date, well-illustrated text represents excellent value for money . . . it's unique in being able to pack so much relevant information into such a small volume, which makes it highly readable"

British Medical Association,
on *Fast Facts – Minor Surgery*, 2nd edn,
(First Prize, Primary Health Care, BMA Book Awards 2008)

"This short textbook provides a quickstop guide to STIs . . . it's handy for both medical students and allied healthcare professionals"

British Medical Association,
on *Fast Facts – Sexually Transmitted Infections*, 2nd edn
(Commended, Public Health Care, BMA Book Awards 2008)

"An outstanding up-to-date compilation of facts on psoriasis, a must-read for any healthcare provider with an interest in psoriasis, whether casual or in-depth"

Dr Gerald Krueger, Professor of Dermatology, University of Utah School of Medicine,
on *Fast Facts – Psoriasis*, 2nd edn, Jan 2009

"A very accessible summary of the key facts about lymphoma, presented in clear language with straightforward explanations"

Leukemia Research Fund,
on *Fast Facts – Lymphoma*, Oct 2008

"A useful addition to this well-known series . . . very affordable and excellent value for money"

ICS News, Feb 2008
on *Fast Facts – Bladder Disorders*

"Buy it for yourself . . . but be careful your colleagues don't borrow it indefinitely"

on *Fast Facts – Asthma*, 2nd edn
Primary Health Care, July 2007

www.fastfacts.com